:60 SECOND
SLEEP-EASE

:60 SECOND
SLEEP-EASE
Quick Tips to Get a Good Night's Rest

Shawn Currie, Ph.D.
and
Keith Wilson, Ph.D.

New Horizon Press
Far Hills, New Jersey

New Horizon Press
P.O. Box 669
Far Hills, NJ 07931

Currie, Shawn and Keith Wilson
   :60 Second Sleep-Ease: Quick Tips to Get a Good Night's Rest

Interior Design: Susan M. Sanderson
Cover Design: Norma Erler Rahn

Library of Congress Catalog Card Number: 2001089196

ISBN: 0-88282-212-8
New Horizon Press

Manufactured in the U.S.A.

2006   2005   2004   2003   2002 / 5   4   3   2   1

AUTHORS' NOTE

The material in this book is intended to provide a quick overview of methods and information now available. Any of the treatments described herein to alleviate sleep disturbances and difficulties should be discussed with a licensed health care practitioner. The authors and publisher assume no responsibility for any adverse outcomes which derive from the use of any of these treatments in a program of self-care or under the care of a licensed practitioner.

The information in this book is based on Shawn Currie's and Keith Wilson's research and practices. Fictitious identities and names have been given to characters in this book, many of whom are composites of patients who participated in the authors' research studies. For the purposes of simplifying usage, the pronouns he and she are often used interchangeably.

TABLE OF CONTENTS

ACKNOWLEDGMENTS

Several individuals assisted in the research studies conducted to evaluate the effectiveness of the material in this book designed to help people suffering from insomnia. They are: Naomi Bodnar, Dr. Stewart Clark, Dorothyann Curran, Lorie deLaplante, Dr. Nady el-Guebaly, Dr. David Hodgins, Andrea Lawson, Nicole Peden, Amanda Pontefract, Stephen Rimac, Joy Robinson and Michelle Shay-Fiddler. Naomi Bodnar also provided invaluable assistance in the preparation of this book. Our research has been supported by the Addiction Centre (Calgary Regional Health Authority) in Calgary, Alberta; Health Canada; the Alberta Heritage Fund for Medical Research; the University of Calgary; the University of Ottawa; the Physical Medical Research Foundation; and the Rehabilitation Centre in Ottawa, Ontario. Finally, we would like to thank the many patients who participated in the clinical trials and provided feedback on the information and advice in this book.

Shawn Currie, Ph.D.
Keith Wilson, Ph.D.

PART 1

SYMPTOMS AND SOURCES
OF INSOMNIA

WHAT CAN YOU DO ABOUT YOUR SLEEP PROBLEMS?: OVERVIEW OF THE :60 SECOND SLEEP-EASE PROGRAM

In this chapter you will:
- *Learn about the :60 second self-management approach for improving sleep*
- *Find out how effective this approach is compared to other sleep treatments*

The :60 Second Self-management Approach for Sleep Problems
Our philosophy of self-management is a simple one. Reading this book is the first 10 percent of the work. This book contains exercises and personal projects for you to try. In a sense, you will become your own therapist and it is up to you to motivate yourself to complete the tasks and use them on a daily basis. You can choose how many you actually try and how often you practice them. The majority of these techniques and exercises can be learned in about :60 seconds; applying them to your sleep will take a little longer. Behavior modification can take several days and in many cases, weeks to yield consistently better sleep. As a word of encouragement, our research shows most people who try these techniques do greatly and rapidly improve their sleep.

The :60 Second program is designed to help you take control of your sleep. Using step-by-step instructions, we will guide you through a series of skills-training exercises and personal projects designed to help you sleep better. One word you will see a lot in this book is "coping." To some people, coping means "just getting by" or surviving a problem. This way of thinking is an example of *passive* coping. Using passive coping strategies during the initial phases of a sleep problem often results in several bad habits being formed. It's easy to fall into a routine of doing nothing about a sleep problem or relying on passive, ineffective ways of coping with your insomnia.

In the :60 Second program, we emphasize a more *active* approach. One way to think of the difference between active and passive coping is to think of the difference between moving forward and staying in one place. When you use passive coping strategies, you stay where you are; your condition may not be getting any worse, but it is also not getting any better. Active coping may involve a little more work on your part in the beginning, but the rewards will be long-term improvement.

An example of passive coping for sleep problems is taking sleeping pills. Initially, they may make you sleep better, but with continued use the effects start to wear off and you have to take more and more of the drug to get the same effects (this is called developing a tolerance to the drug). Eventually, you reach a point where you're taking the maximum dosage allowed—or worse, more than the maximum recommended dosage—and seeing no measurable improvement in your sleep.

Comparison of the :60 Second Self-management Approach and Sleeping Pills

Take :60 seconds to look at Appendix D (page 183), which compares the self-management approach for chronic insomnia to treatment of insomnia with sleeping pills. There are pros and cons to both treatment approaches. For acute or "transient" insomnia, sleeping pills do have a couple of advantages over a self-management or psychological approach since they work very quickly and do not require any real effort on your part. Troublesome side effects, diminishing effectiveness and the expense are the biggest drawbacks to using pills in the treatment of transient insomnia.

For the long-term treatment of chronic insomnia, however, sleeping pills do more harm than good. Sleeping pills are not intended to be taken for months or years at a time. The prolonged use of sleeping pills usually results in a continuing sleep problem and the increased risk of addiction. For chronic insomnia, the self-management approach is much better.

Benefits from this Program

The :60 Second program described in this manual is meant for people with troubling sleep problems for whom long-term treatment with drugs is neither a realistic nor an acceptable option. People who begin this program are generally at the point where they feel they have little or no control over their sleep. The people who will benefit most from the :60 Second program are those who are willing to change the ways they think about sleep and motivated to work toward good sleep goals. Achieving success means a fair amount of work and commitment for individuals. In addition to reading this book, personal projects in the form of exercises will be suggested in each chapter.

What Are You Doing Now to Cope with Your Sleep Problems?

Whether they were homemade or professionally-suggested methods, you have probably tried a variety of things in the past to alleviate your sleep problem. What are some of the things you have tried? Check any of the following that apply.

_____	Sleeping pills	_____	Warm milk
_____	Alcohol	_____	Avoiding caffeine
_____	Relaxation methods	_____	Napping
_____	Over-the-counter sleep aids	_____	Other drugs

The next question is, "How much success have you had with these methods?" If you are like most people, you probably had limited, short term success with some of them, but found that they didn't work on a consistent basis in the long run. A few of the methods on the list *are* valid remedies for disturbed sleep and we will be discussing how you can use them along with other new strategies. In contrast, some of the strategies on this list can actually make your sleep problems worse (alcohol, for example).

Don't worry if you are beginning this program having tried many things in the past—this can actually work to your advantage. For starters, you are probably ready to try something new and different from the other types of treatments which have failed. With the passage of time, you have no doubt become an expert on your own sleep problems and you are probably aware of many factors that can affect your sleep. However, you may not have been given much direction on how to change your sleep habits for consistent improvement. In this book, we encourage you to look at the big picture...that is, how you want your sleep to change over the long-term.

Is the :60 Second Program Effective?
The answer is yes. The program described in this manual combines a variety of effective procedures for the treatment of insomnia. In our practice we have found that each of these strategies has proven helpful for people with chronic sleep problems.

The :60 Second approach you will learn is *evidence-based,* meaning that each of the techniques has proven to work in well-controlled research studies. Our research has shown that combining several different treatment strategies can be even more effective than relying on any one method. This is because different people respond to different types of techniques. By using a variety of techniques, the chances of your sleep improving are greater. In addition, complex sleeping problems usually require more than one strategy. For example, you may have difficulties falling asleep and you may also wake up many times throughout the night. There are specific techniques you can use for coping with each of these problems. This is why it is important for you to try all the strategies in this book and find the combination that works the best for you.

There are, of course, no guaranteed miracle cures. However, about 75 percent of people suffering from chronic sleep problems will experience relief and better sleep using the :60 Second program. This rate of improvement also applies to older adults and to people who have sleep problems because of painful medical conditions. We have conducted research using this treatment on persons with long-standing pain and the elderly and found that their progress in easing sleep difficulties was as good as that seen in primary insomniacs.

How much improvement can you expect? If you use the :60 Second strategies and guidelines as outlined in this book, you should experience a *noticeable improvement* in your sleep, yet the amount really depends on you. The saying "You only get out what you put in" definitely applies to the :60 Second treatment.

Individuals who show the most improvement are those who consistently apply the techniques as they are outlined in the coming chapters. Some people may even become "normal" sleepers. Ultimately, followers of the program will have more satisfying sleep patterns by the time they finish this book. In general, it is more useful to focus on bettering your sleep rather than trying to become a "perfect" sleeper.

Moreover, continuing to use the skills you learn with this program, the progress you make with your sleep can be maintained indefinitely. Our research has shown that improvements made during the course of our self-management program for insomnia are superior to those obtained from the long-term use of sleeping pills. In fact, the prolonged use of sleeping pills usually leads to an eventual worsening of sleep.

What Are the Costs?
The :60 Second program doesn't involve any drugs or special diets. There are no sleep aids or special equipment that you are expected to buy. The only expenses involved are the price of a few pencils, some photocopying and the personal costs of time, energy and motivation. It is vitally important that you do the projects and exercises provided in the coming chapters. This cannot be emphasized enough. Remember that old habits are sometimes hard to break and you must develop new skills.

The Best Way to Use This Book
You will be introduced to and guided through the complete :60 Second self-management approach for coping with chronic sleep problems. Each chapter will begin with an outline of the learning goals for the chapter and a discussion of the rationale for the specific strategies to be practiced. You will then be provided with detailed step-by-step instructions on how to apply the strategies to help you improve your sleep.

Part I of this book analyzes why and how sleep problems occur. Part II is structured to teach behavioral strategies—things to do about your bedtime routine—so that you can immediately begin acquiring the skills that will help you correct your sleeping pattern. Most people will experience improvement in their sleep within the first couple of weeks if they follow these behavioral strategies carefully.

Part III focuses on cognitive skills—methods to change the way you think and feel about sleep-related problems. In these chapters, you will explore the various ways that your thoughts can affect your sleeping behavior and how relaxation exercises can help put your mind at rest.

In Part IV we discuss the special concerns of women, children and adolescents in achieving restful sleep.

As we move to conclusion, Part V reviews various drugs and foods that can affect your sleep. Guidelines are provided on things you should avoid. We will explore the effects of various environmental factors on your sleep and the importance of physical activity.

The final chapter of the book discusses ways in which you can maintain the progress you achieve as a result of the program. Tips on how to incorporate the skills you have learned into your daily routine, information on how to prevent relapses and strategies that can be used to deal with "bad nights" when they occur are offered.

In the appendices will be found sleep resources, a quiz to test your newly acquired knowledge, a sleep log and progress charts for you to evaluate yourself.

Setting Goals and Having Realistic Expectations

Goal-setting should reflect what you would like to get out of the program, as well as how you would like to take permanent control of your sleep. Before you set your goals, you must decide how much of a lifestyle change you are prepared to make. This is by no means a small decision. Remember that you spend almost one-third of your life in bed, so you are making a commitment to alter a substantial portion of your life. If you are ready to make this decision, then the rest of the program should proceed smoothly.

:60 Second Guidelines for Setting Goals

Setting realistic goals involves both creativity and some common sense. Use the following criteria to set your goals.

Criteria (A goal should be...)	Something to ask	A well-defined goal	A poorly-defined goal
Measurable	How will you evaluate the goal when it has been reached?	I want to be able to fall asleep within thirty minutes at least five nights per week.	I want to have more REM sleep.
Realistic	Is the goal within your grasp?	I want to have one less awakening each night.	I want to sleep eight hours straight every night of the week.
Specific	Does achieving it involve specific actions to take?	I want to cut out daytime napping.	I want to sleep better.
"I"-centered	Are you the one taking the actions to be measured?	I will try to do thirty minutes of exercise daily.	I want a better sleeping pill.

If you are having a hard time coming up with some goals, you can try the following :60 Second exercise. Long before you started this program, you probably had the desire to sleep better. Maybe you expressed this desire in an "I wish" statement (e.g., "I wish I could sleep through the night without waking up so often"). Think back to some of your desires and wish statements and then complete the following "I wish" sentences with statements concerning your sleep.

I wish _____.
I wish _____.
I wish _____.

Now, look at your "I wish" statements. Do they meet the goal-setting criteria? If possible, modify and rewrite the goals that don't meet all the criteria. Consider making goals smaller as a means of making them more realistic. Wanting to fall asleep within five minutes of going to bed is probably unrealistic. Remember that most people without insomnia can't fall asleep within five minutes. Rather, if it now takes you an hour to fall asleep, consider setting a goal of being able to fall asleep within thirty minutes.

An important thing to keep in mind is that there is nothing wrong with an occasional setback when trying to make a permanent behavior change. Later in the program, we will talk about setbacks in more detail and ways of dealing with them without getting discouraged. Let's begin by finding out just what insomnia and normal sleep are, the causes of chronic insomnia and why you can't get that good night's sleep you crave.

chapter 2

CHRONIC INSOMNIA

In this chapter you will learn:
- *Signs and consequences of insomnia*
- *How to assess your insomnia*
- *Other sleep disorders and when to seek professional help*

Signs of Chronic Insomnia

If you're reading this book, you must be having some trouble sleeping. You may even have had sleep problems for years. If so, you are certainly not alone. Millions of people struggle with insomnia and other problems caused by a lack of proper rest each night. Here is a checklist of the most common symptoms of insomnia. Mark off those symptoms that have bothered you for more than one month.

:60 Second Sleepless Checklist

_____Trouble falling asleep

_____Trouble staying asleep (waking up through the night)

_____Feeling tired during the day

_____Waking up earlier in the morning than you would like to

_____Feeling irritable or depressed during the day

_____Feeling that your sleep is unrefreshing and of poor quality

_____Falling asleep in inappropriate places (e.g., at work)

These are the classic symptoms of insomnia. Almost everyone experiences insomnia at some time during his or her life. Unfortunately, it seems to strike at the most inconvenient times—the night before an important interview, during a period of sickness or when your baby has finally started to sleep through the night. Usually, insomnia is brought on by a period of high stress or after a major life change. The variety of problems that constitute insomnia are considered to be situational and they are usually time-limited, lasting only a few days or a couple of weeks. Situational or occasional insomnia usually clears up in a short time. When the situation improves and life seems normal again, the insomnia seems to go away. For occasional insomnia, one good night's sleep is all one usually needs to snap out of it. However, insomnia can also appear out of the blue with no clear-cut problems that seem to bring it on.

When sleep difficulties last for more than one month, we consider the person to have a problem with chronic insomnia. Although chronic insomnia is not as common in the general population as occasional insomnia, it usually causes far more problems in an individual's life. This book was written primarily for people with chronic insomnia, although anyone who has ever had problems sleeping will probably find helpful information and advice in the coming chapters.

How Common is Insomnia?

The short answer to this question is *very* common. Surveys conducted over the last twenty years have shown the rate of chronic insomnia in the adult population to be fairly stable at about 10 percent or about twenty-five million people.[1] About one-third of Americans, for instance, report that they have occasional problems sleeping. The rates in other industrialized countries are about the same. A 1991 survey found that people with occasional insomnia had an average of five nights of poor sleep each month. In comparison, chronic insomniacs had an average of sixteen bad nights in a typical month. The most common complaint of both occasional and chronic insomniacs was waking up feeling unrefreshed. Over half of the insomniacs surveyed also reported problems getting to sleep and staying asleep.

Insomnia is a more common complaint among women, although a greater number of men are thought to underreport or deny the problem. It may be that women are more open than men to admitting to problems with their health and well-being. One researcher has even suggested that women have more sleep problems, because they spend much of their lives trying to sleep beside men who snore!

Despite being such a widespread problem, the availability of treatment for insomnia is limited. Surprisingly few insomniacs ever talk to physicians or other health professionals about their sleep problems. In one telephone survey, two-thirds of the insomniacs questioned indicated that they knew very little about the treatment options for their sleep problems. This leads us to believe that many insomniacs suffer in silence. Those who do seek medical treatment are most likely to be prescribed sleeping pills over other forms of treatment. However, only about half of chronic insomniacs find sleep medications helpful. Most sleep experts agree that medication should be avoided for persons with chronic sleep problems due to the risk of drug dependence and side effects that may result in impairment of daytime functioning. Nevertheless, the chronic insomniacs surveyed were on medication for an average of two years, with many reporting that they took sleeping pills for over ten years. Many insomniacs resort to various self-help treatments to try to improve their sleep. For example, almost one-third of Americans with insomnia report using alcohol to help them sleep. The deleterious effects of medications and alcohol on sleep will be discussed in more detail in later chapters.

What Problems Does Insomnia Cause?

Persistent sleep problems cause many difficulties, both on personal and societal levels. Compared to good sleepers, insomniacs are twice as likely to get into motor vehicle accidents. One of the reasons for some large-scale industrial accidents (Three Mile Island and Chernobyl, for example), has been attributed to worker fatigue during night shifts. In addition to the risk of accidents, chronic insomniacs are much more vulnerable to mental health problems like depression and anxiety. They may feel unproductive at work because of problems concentrating and feelings of fatigue during the day. In a recent study, insomniacs questioned estimated that they were working at about three-quarters of their usual capacities.[2] They attributed their reduced productivity to problems attending to instructions, being irritable around co-workers and having trouble making decisions.

Although daytime impairment is commonly associated with poor sleep, it should be noted that recent thinking is that these problems may not be directly caused by sleep loss. In controlled lab experiments, volunteers appear to cope reasonably well after being completely deprived of sleep for two or three nights in a row. They show some deficits on repetitive tasks that require prolonged concentration, but do well on tasks that are more complicated and interesting.[3] Most people can recover their lost sleep in a relatively short period of time—a few hours in fact. Many experts now believe that daytime problems that are reported by people with occasional or short-term insomnia are due in large part to the original problems that led to their sleep difficulties. For example, people who are not sleeping well because they are having marital problems is likely to be irritable and distracted during the day because of their preoccupation with their personal crises. Preoccupation with sleep loss itself can cause issues during the day. If you don't sleep well and convince yourself you will have a bad day because of it, you are setting yourself up to be miserable. The role of thoughts and beliefs in sleep problems is discussed in more detail in chapter 10, along with techniques for changing sleep-interfering thoughts.

Though some perceptions about sleep deprivation are ill-founded, it is true that chronic insomnia can lower one's resistance to stress related and physical illnesses. Health difficulties like headaches, stomach problems and back pain are more common in persons with chronic insomnia. Determining cause and effect is difficult, because many medical problems like chronic pain are also a cause of sleep problems. Assessing which came first is often impossible. Many insomniacs report they have had sleep problems their entire lives. They often have hard times identifying what was going on when their sleep problems started. Even if their insomnia eventually gets worse and they develop other health problems on top of it, their memories of what triggered the original sleeplessness are scanty. Regardless of the original cause, it is generally believed that insomnia is perpetuated or worsened by psychological factors even when there may be physical health problems that are part of the initial cause. The combination of health problems, emotional stress and feeling tired during the day can take a great toll on individuals with serious sleep problems. Quality of life can suffer tremendously[4] and the ability to cope with new life stressors is often diminished.

The economic costs of insomnia to society have been estimated by researchers pooling information from different sources on health care expenses.[5] For example, data collected in 1995 revealed that over $800 million in the United States was spent on prescription sleeping pills and another $350 million was spent on non-prescription (over-the-counter) sleep aids. Based on the number of people who claim to use alcohol to help them fall asleep, an estimated $780 million is spent every year on alcohol for its use as a sleep aid. In 1994, there were over eight million physician visits because of sleep complaints. This cost individuals and insurance companies who were paying about $660 million. Another $260 million was spent on trips to psychologists, social workers and sleep specialists for help with insomnia. We could also add the cost of nursing home care. Over 60 percent of caregivers report their elderly relatives' sleep disturbances as a contributing factor in choosing institutionalization. Put it all together and insomnia is thought to cost about ten billion dollars per year in America alone. Worldwide, the cost is many times this amount.

It is important to note that many of these costs are based on the number of people who actually seek help. More than half of insomnia sufferers never seek professional help and less than 1 percent get help from sleep specialists. The costs could be much higher if all insomniacs sought treatment. Furthermore, the indirect costs of insomnia in terms of chronic absenteeism and reduced work productivity are unknown, but are estimated to be substantial.

:60 Second Self-assessment

Sleep specialists use a variety of methods to assess your sleep and diagnose insomnia. By far the most common method is the sleep log. If you go to a sleep clinic, you are likely to be given this assessment log to complete every morning for a week or two. In the log you will keep track of your sleep habits, such as the time you go to bed, how long it takes you to fall asleep and the quality of your sleep. Contrary to what some people believe, it is usually not necessary to stay overnight in a sleep lab to diagnose insomnia. Sleep disorder clinics usually do not recommend an overnight sleep evaluation unless you exhibit symptoms of other sleep disorders like sleep apnea, a serious medical condition characterized by abnormal breathing during sleep (discussed in greater detail later in this chapter). Ironically, many insomniacs actually sleep better in sleep labs, because they are away from their usual sleepless environments.

The best way to diagnose your problem is to complete the sleep log provided in chapter 5 and Appendix C for a couple of weeks to get a current record of your sleep pattern. For now, you can complete the following :60 Second self-assessment questionnaire based on how your sleep has been in the last two months.

:60 Second Sleep Assessment Quiz

1. a. In a typical week, are there nights when it takes you more than thirty minutes to fall asleep?

    _____Yes _____No

    b. If you answered yes, how many nights in a typical week does this happen?

    _____Once

    _____Twice

    _____Three times or more

2. a. In a typical week, are there nights when you wake up through the night and have trouble getting back to sleep?

    _____Yes _____No

    b. If you answered yes, how many nights in a typical week does this happen?

    _____Once

    _____Twice

    _____Three times or more

3. a. In a typical week, are there mornings when you wake up ear-
    lier than you wanted to and have trouble getting back to sleep?
    _____Yes _____No

    b. If you answered yes, how many mornings in a typical week
    does this happen?
    _____Once
    _____Twice
    _____Three times or more

4. a. In a typical week, do you wake up feeling like your sleep was
    not restful?
    _____Yes _____No

    b. If you answered yes, how many nights in a typical week does
    this happen?
    _____Once
    _____Twice
    _____Three times or more

5. Do you feel your sleep problem is a direct cause of:
    _____significant distress for you
    _____missing time at work
    _____not doing your job well when at work
    _____missing social functions
    _____problems getting along with friends, family or co-workers

6. Have your sleep difficulties been going on for more than one
    month?
    _____Yes _____No

    If you answered yes to questions 1, 2, 3 or 4, and indicated
that your sleep problem happens three times per week or more for at
least one of these questions, then you do indeed have some significant symptoms of insomnia. If you checked off at least one of the
problems listed in question 5 and indicated on question 6 that this has

been going on for more than one month, then there is a good chance you have an insomnia *disorder*. A disorder means that the insomnia symptoms are severe enough to cause problems in your life.

If your sleep problem does not meet these criteria above (for example, you have trouble falling asleep, but only once or twice per week), the reason could be that you have only mild or occasional insomnia. This is good news, because it means your sleep problems are likely not bad enough to cause you tremendous difficulties in your day-to-day life. Nevertheless, the information and coping strategies in this book can still be helpful to you. Persons with mild or occasional insomnia should still follow the recommendations for good sleep habits in the coming chapters. Chapter 7, for example, will show you how to be a good sleeper all the time. By doing something now about your minor sleep problems, you may possibly prevent a mild insomnia condition from becoming chronic.

If you rated yourself as having an insomnia disorder, follow the advice provided in the next chapters. Knowing that you have an insomnia disorder does not tell anything about the cause of the insomnia problem. The first step is to have a complete physical examination. Generally, if you are in good health, not experiencing any significant emotional problems (apart from those caused by insomnia) and don't have any of the symptoms of the other sleep disorders discussed in the next section, you probably have *primary* insomnia. This means your insomnia is not being caused by a physical problem.

In contrast, a person with *secondary* insomnia has sleep difficulties that are mainly caused by a medical or psychological problem. For example, sleep disturbances can be a symptom of depression. Insomnia symptoms can also be the result of other sleep disorders, as you will read later in this chapter. In most cases, persons with secondary insomnia can still benefit from the techniques in this book.

Types of Insomnia
There are three main types of insomnia. They are classified on the basis of the portion of the night (beginning, middle or end) in which sleep is most disturbed. People whose primary difficulty is falling asleep are called *sleep onset insomniacs*. Those who have problems

staying asleep are considered to have *sleep maintenance insomnia*. Finally, individuals who are able sleep through the night but wake up two hours or more before their desired arising time have *early morning awakenings*. In reality most insomnia patients experience a combination of these problems. It is also not uncommon for the type of insomnia to fluctuate over time.

There are :60 Second techniques in this book to help you with each of these problems. Because most people have a combination of sleep onset and maintenance problems, try all the strategies and find the ones that work best for you.

Other Sleep Disorders

Medical diagnostic textbooks list over a dozen sleep disorders. By far the most common are the insomnia disorders (primary and secondary). Sleep apnea is the next most common sleep disorder. Sleep apnea is a serious medical condition that is caused by the cessation of airflow through the mouth and nose during sleep. People with sleep apnea generally breath normally during the day, so many don't know they have it. At night, however, they may stop breathing between 200 and 500 times, causing frequent disruption of their sleep. Some people with severe apnea are lucky to get five minutes of uninterrupted sleep. The causes of sleep apnea can be anatomical (an actual obstruction in the airway during sleep), neurological or a combination of the two. There are several telling signs of sleep apnea along with various risk factors. The most common symptoms are:

- Snoring loudly
- Pauses in breathing while you sleep
- Waking up with a dry mouth every morning
- Waking up with a headache almost every morning
- Feeling extremely tired during the day

You may not be aware of the first two symptoms unless you have a bed partner who has complained that you snore or wake up gasping for breath several times through the night. There are also several risk factors for sleep apnea. Men are more susceptible than women. Lifestyle factors like smoking, regular alcohol use, being

overweight and high blood pressure can increase the risk. If you suspect you may have sleep apnea, you should talk to your doctor immediately. He or she will arrange a referral to a sleep clinic where you can
be properly assessed. The sleep clinic will probably have you stay
overnight in the laboratory so that your breathing and brain activity
during sleep can be measured. Fortunately, there are several effective
treatments for this disorder. Surgery can help to clear any obstruction
in your airway. Many patients buy or rent a machine that provides continuous positive airway pressure (CPAP) and keeps your airway open
while you sleep. Losing weight is also recommended if you are
severely overweight and quitting smoking is always a good idea.
Finally, the techniques provided in this book can help you get your
sleep pattern back on track.

   Restless legs syndrome and *periodic limb movements* are two related
sleep disorders that appear less frequently in adults than sleep apnea.
The symptoms of restless legs syndrome include:

- Unpleasant, crawling, aching sensation in your calves during
  the day and in bed at night
- Irresistible urge to move your legs in bed
- Worsening symptoms when sitting down and at night

   Most people with restless legs syndrome also have periodic
limb movements. The primary symptom of this disorder is having
brief repetitive movements (twitches or jerks) of the legs during sleep.
Many people are not aware they are making these movements and
only find out when their bed partner complains that he or she is being
kicked throughout the night. Restless legs syndrome usually causes
problems getting to sleep while periodic limb movements may lead to
problems staying asleep. Both of these conditions seem to worsen
with age. This may be due to an age-related decline of blood circula-
tion in the limbs, which is one of the suspected causes of both conditions. Treatment can include medications that relax the muscles and
vitamin supplements to adjust for deficiencies in various vitamins and
minerals.

Most of the remaining sleep disorders are extremely rare—narcolepsy, for example—while some others primarily occur in children, such as sleepwalking, which is discussed in chapter 13. If you suspect you have a sleep disorder other than insomnia, you should talk to your doctor right away and request a referral to a sleep clinic (you may have to travel out of town if there is not one in your area). A list of resources on other sleep disorders is provided in Appendix A.

chapter 3

CAUSES OF INSOMNIA

In this chapter you will learn:
* *How chronic insomnia often starts and is maintained over time*
* *About the medical and psychological causes of insomnia*

What Causes Insomnia?

Insomnia, unlike many other disorders, is not caused by a single factor or event. Rather, the chronic inability to sleep is thought to be caused by a constellation of factors that is different for every person. Foremost, insomnia is often a symptom of another problem. Persons with medical conditions that involve pain or some form of discomfort are likely to have sleep problems. Psychiatric problems like major depression and many anxiety disorders, as well as emotional problems, can also cause sleep disturbances. Very often, resolution of the under-lying problems will result in the sleep problems also improving. On the other hand, this doesn't always happen. Insomnia typically starts during a period of high stress (for example, during a divorce, after getting fired from a job, etc.), but can continue despite the original stressor going away or being resolved. There are several possible reasons for this fail-ure of a sleep problem to fade away along with its initial cause.

First, during the period of stress the insomniac may come to associate the bed and bedroom with sleeplessness. Many people can function well during the day, because they have things to take their mind off the stress—work or household chores, for example. At night, however, escaping the negative emotions brought on by the stress is more difficult. You may begin to dread going to bed because you know that you will be alone with difficult thoughts and opportunities to ruminate about the problems you are facing. Your bed can actually become a signal or "trigger" for poor sleep. Your bed and bedroom should be places that promote a sense of calm restfulness. However, if you get into the habit of lying in bed for long periods with "racing thoughts," your bed and bedroom can begin to promote anxious wakefulness instead. This process is called *conditioning* and is discussed in chapter 7.

Second, many coping strategies people try for their insomnia end up making their sleep problems worse. Here are a few big mistakes that are commonly made by people with insomnia:

- Going to bed earlier or sleeping in later in the morning in the hopes of recovering lost sleep. This results in spending more and more time in bed not sleeping, thereby reinforcing the bed as a trigger for insomnia.
- Napping during the day. This provides temporary relief from feeling tired, but can make nighttime sleep worse.
- Falling asleep in places other than the bed—while watching television, for example—which does not help build a positive association between the bed and sleeping.
- Drinking large amounts of coffee to keep alert during the day, drinking alcohol at night to fall asleep or both.
- Reducing physical activity because of feelings of fatigue and becoming more and more sedentary.
- Starting to rely on external sleep aids like prescription sleeping pills or over-the-counter sleep aids.

Finally, sleep-disturbed people may start to obsess about their sleep problems. They might have catastrophic thoughts about never sleeping well again. They may come to believe the only way to get more sleep is to take medications or drink alcohol. Simply going to bed may bring on anxiety, making sleep even less likely. Insomniacs frequently develop their own version of *performance anxiety*, so that the actual process of trying to fall asleep ends up stirring the opposite reaction: apprehension, arousal, tension and, ultimately, frustration.

Does any of this sound familiar? Other telling signs that your sleep problem is at least partly due to learned poor sleep habits are:

- Starting to feel tense when getting ready for bed (getting undressed, brushing your teeth).
- Worrying, as bedtime approaches, whether you will be able to sleep well.
- Sleeping better in unfamiliar settings, like staying at a friend's house or on the bus.
- Experiencing sleep problems even when the original stress event is gone or much improved.

When the cause of disturbed sleep is identified as a medical or psychological problem, most sleep experts agree that treating the underlying condition should take priority over treatment of the insomnia. There are times, however, when direct treatment of a sleep problem can be beneficial even if the original cause of the sleep problem has not gone away. Persons with chronic pain, for example, will often reach limits with what medical treatments can do for them and they may want to try self-management approaches to help improve their sleep. At some point, further medical treatments can actually worsen pain problems. Some medical advice can also make sleep problems worse—for example, advising ongoing bed rest and prescribing numerous medications at once. Depressed individuals can benefit from the behavioral strategies in chapters 6 and 7 if their depressions are no longer severe. In fact, exerting control over one's insomnia can be therapeutic for a person who is still feeling pessimistic about things in general. Focusing on sleep for a while can increase an individual's sense of control over his or her environment, which in turn can improve depression.

Good Versus Bad Sleepers

Many patients say, "I have always been a bad sleeper. There is nothing I can do." Viewing yourself as either a good or bad sleeper is an example of inflexible thinking (this will be discussed in more detail in chapter 10). The reality is that all "good" sleepers have periods of insomnia and most chronic insomniacs (the "bad" sleepers) still have some good nights. Hence, the distinction between a good and bad sleeper is not that clear. Nevertheless, research conducted on insomniacs during the last thirty years has provided sleep experts with a better profile of a person who is likely to have persistent sleep problems. In addition, it has been noted that women are more at risk to develop chronic insomnia. Also, some people are more prone to chronic physiological arousal. They have harder times relaxing and winding down when they want to sleep. These people may feel more tense and hyperactive during the day. They usually react to stress with greater physical and psychological responses. One would expect such people to burn out by the evening, be tired and ready for rest when bedtime comes around. Instead, they typically feel physically exhausted in the evening, but their minds are still racing. The onset of sleep is usually delayed, because these individuals have hard times turning their thoughts off.

This kind of chronic overaroused state may be partly due to hereditary factors. Many people are born with anxiety-prone temperaments. Consequently, many chronic adult insomniacs had sleep problems as children. Their parents will usually recall that it was difficult to get them to sleep at night. Often insomnia runs in families. If you have it, ask members of your family if they do. Chances are you are not the only one. Like most traits, however, only part of insomnia can be blamed on genetics. Environmental factors are equally if not more important. You may have grown up in a house of chronic worriers who tended to get anxious over the smallest of problems. Growing up in a noisy home where people worked odd hours and kept irregular sleeping habits can also contribute to developing chronic insomnia as an adult.

Sleep problems are more common among people who are divorced, widowed or separated and among persons with low income. The common denominator unifying these groups of people is high levels of stress. Certain personality traits are also associated with chronic insomnia. People who describe themselves as chronic worriers and who tend to obsess about problems, even minor ones, are prone to insomnia. Individuals who have low self-esteem and get easily depressed are at risk. Many such people tend to experience various physical symptoms in addition to psychological problems.

We have discussed how insomnia is very often a learned condition. Although some people are more predisposed to get chronic insomnia, they still have to learn how to be bad sleepers over time. Many insomniacs report that their sleep problems began early in life, often around the time of significant stress events, but then worsened over time. This is usually because such peoples' attempts to cope with sleep problems made them worse or at least kept the problems from getting better on their own.

Chronic Pain and Insomnia

One of the more common sources of insomnia is chronic pain. One national survey conducted in Canada found that 44 percent of adults who had some kind of painful medical condition also reported serious sleep disturbances.[1] There are many types of chronic pain conditions. People with chronic back or neck pains seem to be most at risk for developing problems sleeping because of the difficulties they experience in finding comfortable positions in bed. The sleep problems of people with chronic pain are nearly identical to those of people with primary insomnia. For example, they have trouble falling asleep, wake up several times at night and feel unrefreshed in the morning. However, persons with chronic pain seem to do a lot more tossing and turning in bed, because they cannot stay in one position for long.

The most common complaint of people with chronic pain is that pain wakes them up. Our research has certainly shown that people with chronic pain have more awakenings than pain-free sleepers. However, it is unlikely that chronic pain could actually wake a person from a sleeping state. Rather, it is thought that people with chronic pain experience generally lighter sleep than pain-free sleepers. Chronic pain sufferers may be more susceptible to being aroused by their external environments (for example, noise or extreme room temperatures). When they reach waking states in their sleep period—which is a normal event for all sleepers—they may become immediately aware of their discomforting pain. Then they go through cycles of shifting several times in attempts to find comfortable positions. In essence, it may be like trying to fall asleep for the first time again. Hence, most people with chronic pain have severe sleep maintenance insomnia.

Another sleep problem people with chronic pain experience is spending excess time in bed. Many people with chronic pain report being able to sleep only four to six hours a night. However, many lie in bed for much longer—sometimes ten hours or more—hoping for more sleep. Because of this, they only spend about 50 percent to 65 percent of their time in bed actually sleeping, in contrast to good sleepers who normally spend about 90 percent of their time in bed sleeping.

Living in constant pain for a long time leads many people to develop poor sleep habits and lifestyles that may ultimately worsen sleep problems. For example, many persons with chronic pain tend to develop rather sedentary lifestyles. They may spend lots of time resting or even napping during the day, usually in bed. Many individuals with severe chronic pain tend to organize a lot of their daytime activities around their bedrooms. As mentioned earlier, these activities can be harmful to sleep because they create a strong association between the bedroom and sleeplessness. Figure 3.1 shows how chronic pain can eventually lead to chronic insomnia for many people.

In addition to the influence of sleep habits, a number of drugs commonly taken by people with chronic pain (for example, aspirin, muscle relaxants and sleeping pills) can disturb normal sleep and suppress the amount of deep sleep attained during the night. Too often people with chronic pain are over-medicated with drugs that do more harm than good in the long term.

All of this may sound discouraging if you are experiencing chronic pain. The good news, however, is that the strategies in this book are also very effective for someone with sleep problems due to pain. Our research and other studies have shown that people with chronic pain who follow the procedures in the coming chapters show large improvements in their sleep.[2] Some even became normal sleepers. Also remember that not everyone with chronic pain has sleep problems and those that do routinely have some good nights of sleep just like people with chronic insomnia. Many factors that contribute to poor sleep can be changed with a little work on your part.

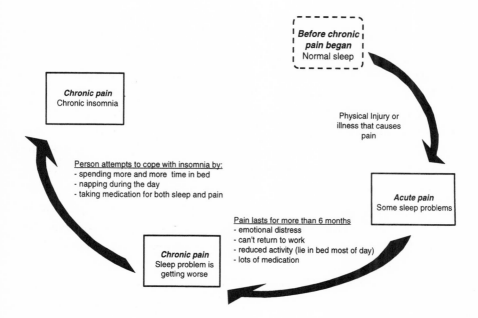

Figure 3.1

Sleep and Alcohol Abuse

Some people use alcohol to get to sleep. In fact, one survey conducted in the United States in 1991 found that more people used alcohol as a sleep aid than medication. Six percent of the population reported using alcohol to fall asleep at least once per week. Despite alcohol's popularity, it is a myth that alcohol improves sleep. It doesn't! While it is true that as a central nervous system depressant, alcohol can induce sleep if a sufficient quantity is consumed, the overall effect is to disturb sleep for a number of reasons. First, alcohol withdrawal will be experienced in the middle of the night as the alcohol is metabolized in the body. Second, alcohol alters the pattern of sleep stage changes, leading to a "short-circuit" of the normal sleep cycle. Third, alcohol increases the frequency of urination, meaning of course, more frequent trips to the bathroom during the night. Finally, alcohol can increase snoring and make breathing difficult for those with pre-existing respiratory problems.

Insomniacs are more likely than good sleepers to develop drinking problems if they use alcohol as a sleep aid on a regular basis. In a recent study, insomniacs and good sleepers were given their choice of two beverages that looked and tasted the same at bedtime. One contained alcohol and the other did not (the subjects did not know which beverage contained the alcohol). When they tried both, the insomniacs chose the beverage containing alcohol more often than the normal sleepers. On a sleep log completed in the morning, the insomniacs reported feeling that the alcohol helped them sleep better, when in fact actual recordings taken overnight showed the alcohol had a more disruptive effect on their sleep in the second half of the night.[3]

This study shows how easy it may be for people with insomnia to believe that alcohol helps them sleep when the opposite is usually true. Unfortunately, the continued use of alcohol as a sleep aid can lead to a vicious cycle of worsening sleep and reliance on alcohol to get to sleep. Research has shown that repeated heavy use of alcohol leads to, among numerous other health problems, chronically poor sleep. Alcohol and substance abuse problems account for more complaints of poor sleep in the general population than do medical disorders. Those with alcohol problems also experience severe sleep disturbances when they stop drinking and go through withdrawal. Although sleep usually improves after a week or two, most alcoholics continue to experience disrupted sleep for many months and even years. Researchers don't quite know why. There are, however, a few plausible explanations. It is possible the brain needs time to heal after long periods of alcohol abuse. We also know that alcoholics tend to have poor sleep *habits* which seem to persist even after they stop drinking.

> *Peter, a self-employed real estate agent, regularly drank eight to ten bottles of beer every night. He went to bed between 1:00 A.M. and 3:00 A.M. and woke up between nine and eleven the*

next morning. He woke up hungover and usually napped in the late afternoon. He began drinking in the evening again. This pattern continued for several years until Peter joined AA and quit drinking. His sleep improved after quitting, but remained light and unrefreshing. He found himself sticking to his old routine of sleeping late and napping later in the day, causing him to be up late in the evening once again.

If you have had a drinking problem in the past, your success with the :60 Second program will be greater if you maintain complete abstinence from alcohol and other drugs (apart from those prescribed for you). Resuming regular drinking will only make your sleep problems worse. Furthermore, the strategies you will learn in this program will help you fall asleep quicker, have fewer awakenings and get a more refreshing sleep.

Insomnia in the Elderly

Over one-half of all persons sixty-five years and older report having some sleep problems and about 20 percent complain of chronic insomnia. For most older adults, their sleep problems resemble the type labeled as sleep maintenance insomnia. Getting to sleep is often not a major problem, but staying asleep is. In the previous chapter we mentioned that sleep difficulties are a major reason why many caregivers choose to put elderly parents or grandparents in nursing homes. Many elderly persons are up several times through the night and can only sleep for continuous periods of time during the day. If you live in a small home, these restless nights can be disruptive and very frustrating to you and other family members trying to sleep.

Sleep problems in the elderly do not start suddenly, although there are predictable milestones that can trigger insomnia. Retirement, for example, is a stressful transition period for most people. The absence of a daily routine can wreak havoc on an individual's sleep schedule. Furthermore, many people become less active in their retirement. However, natural changes in sleep patterns start long before retirement. For most of us, our sleep begins to show a change in our thirties.[4] We begin to get less deep sleep, with the most pronounced change in sleep patterns seen in our early sixties. Between the ages of thirty and sixty, most people begin to notice that they have more awakenings and that they are getting less sleep at night. This biological fact is often taken to mean that older people *need* less sleep. However, it is a misperception that we need less sleep as we get older. Some older adults find they sleep less during the night, but start napping during the day. Hence, the total amount of sleep may not change; it is simply redistributed around the twenty-four-hour clock. Many older people still spend about the same amount of time in bed at night, despite sleeping less. Consequently, they have very inefficient and light sleep. Getting up in the morning, they recall their night's sleep as being poor and may nap during the day in an attempt to compensate.

Several other factors can contribute to sleep problems for mature adults. Health problems start to accumulate as people get older. The pain associated with arthritis, for example, can be a distraction while lying in bed awaiting sleep. An increase in respiratory problems (chronic cough, emphysema) is associated with aging. The rate of sleep apnea problems increases with age, particularly in men. Another medical problem that affects many men as they grow older is enlargement of the prostate gland, which puts more pressure on the bladder (women experience something similar during pregnancy). This results in *nocturia,* or frequent urination during the night. Getting up to urinate several times during the night can be very disruptive to the sleep pattern, especially when you are already not getting much deep sleep. Your body starts to get used to the multiple awakenings through the night, leading you to feel your sleep is constantly being disrupted.

Many elderly persons take medications for a variety of reasons, including sleep problems. About 10 percent to 15 percent of adults over fifty-five in the United States take sleeping pills, many for several years. As you will read in chapter 8, long-term use of these medications can impair sleep more than enhance it. Most sleeping pills reduce the amount of deep sleep, which is particularly problematic for individuals who already have reduced deep sleep periods because they are older. Pain medications can also disrupt sleep. Psychological problems like depression are common in the elderly. Many older adults face a number of losses as they age: loss of regular employment through retirement, loss of spouses and friends, isolation from family, etc. These stressors can add up and the combined effect is often overwhelming, causing troubled sleep.

The news is not completely bad, however. Lots of older people have no sleep problems at all. There are many people in their seventies, eighties and even nineties who report that their quality of sleep is the same as people half their age. If an older individual does have chronic insomnia, he or she does not have to feel powerless about it. Many of the factors that contribute to poor sleep can be changed. It is a myth that the only treatment for insomnia in the elderly is medication. In fact, Dr. Charles Morin and his colleagues at Virginia Commonwealth University conducted a study that compared a non-drug treatment (similar to the one proposed in this book) to a common sleeping pill in the treatment of late-life insomnia.[5] Not only did the non-drug method work as well as the medication, it resulted in a longer-lasting improvement in sleep, which was confirmed by the patients when they were seen six and twelve months after the treatment was completed.

This means that a non-drug treatment is more likely to produce long-term change. This makes sense when one considers that a behavioral treatment for insomnia generally gets to the roots of the problem, which are correcting bad sleep habits and teaching patients how to control their insomnia. The skills that you can learn to improve your sleep are skills that you will have for the rest of your life. Sleeping pills may be helpful at first, but in the long run they can actually contribute to ongoing sleep problems. Unfortunately, persons over fifty-five are the largest segment of the population for whom sedative medication is prescribed.

chapter 4

NORMAL SLEEP

In this chapter you will learn:
* *The biological aspects of sleep*
* *The function sleep serves*

What Happens to Your Brain When You Sleep?

To benefit fully from the :60 Second program, it is important to have some basic information on sleep. It is a misconception that sleep is a "passive" event. In fact, your body and mind are hard at work when you sleep. For example, dreaming that occurs mostly during REM sleep is a very active state of the mind. REM stands for Rapid Eye Movement, which describes the activity of your eyes during this stage of sleep. REM sleep is only one stage of sleep. There are a total of five stages in human sleep. The other four stages are simply referred to as Stages 1 to 4. These are collectively referred to as the "non-REM" stages of sleep.

The stages are numbered to indicate progressively "deeper" sleep; Stage 1 is the lightest form of sleep while Stage 4 is the deepest. Stage 1 is actually very light sleep. A person in this stage can be awakened more easily than during deep or REM sleep stages. Sleep of stages 3 and 4 is referred to as deep sleep or *slow-wave* sleep, which is the technical name for the slow, low frequency brain waves observed during these stages. During deep sleep, a person is quite still and breathes very slowly. It is very difficult to wake someone up from deep sleep. Given its importance, several references will be made to deep sleep throughout this book. We will discuss, for example, ways that you might be able to increase your nighttime deep sleep.

As you are now aware, the process of sleeping is not like turning a switch ON or OFF. There are several stages to sleep and these stages differ in terms of their depth and length. You might now wonder how your body organizes all these different sleep stages. It is actually not that complicated. Your body cycles through the five stages of sleep in intervals of approximately ninety minutes in length (see below). You can use the occurrence of REM sleep as a marker for the beginning of this cycle. Thus, every ninety minutes or so, you enter the REM, or dreaming, stage of sleep. The amount of time spent in the different stages depends on many factors such as age, activity level and sleep history. For a normal young adult with no sleep problems, the breakdown is something like:

- Awake, about 5% of the night
- Stage 1, about 5% of the night
- Stage 2, about 50% of the night
- Deep sleep (Stages 3 and 4), about 20% of the night
- REM sleep, about 20% of the night

An important thing to know about the sleep cycle is that throughout the night, a person actually reaches a waking state several times. That is, it is quite normal for someone to experience awakenings during the night. In fact, the average adult has between fifteen to twenty brief awakenings or arousals every night. Most of these arousals are not full awakenings and only last a few seconds. People do not generally remember awakening during the night unless they open their eyes, wake up from a bad dream or get up to go to the bathroom.

There is much more about the biology of sleep that could be discussed, but it is not essential to this program. What is critical is that you are familiar with the terms *deep sleep*, *awakening* and *sleep cycle*, because they will become important in subsequent chapters.

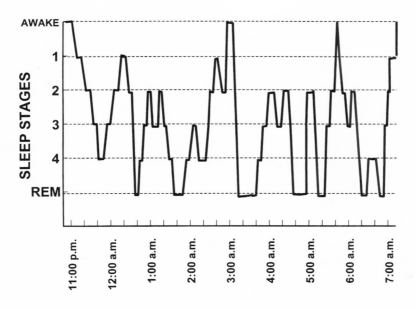

TIME OF NIGHT

Figure 4.1. This graph shows how your brain cycles through the five stages of sleep during the night. Although this is a simplified version of what actually happens, it shows roughly the percentage of time spent in the sleep stages. Rapid eye movement (REM) sleep is more concentrated in the last part of the sleep period.

Why Do We Need to Sleep?

We spend almost one third of our lives sleeping, so it is no wonder that quality sleep is important. No doubt everyone is aware that sleep is hardly a voluntary process. Although we may have some control in prolonging the onset of sleep (e.g., staying up late to watch a good movie), one way or another, we eventually need to sleep.

People differ in the amount of sleep they require to function adequately. Although the average for healthy adults is about seven to eight hours per night, the range of sleep time that people find refreshing is between four to twelve hours per night. About 20 percent of the adult population sleep six hours or less a night. Thus, the notions of "oversleeping" or not getting enough sleep are highly personal. For example, a person who habitually sleeps five hours per night and then gets eight hours of sleep on one particular night may actually feel that he or she has overslept. How we grew up has a big impact on our sleep needs as adults. For example, if you grew up on a farm and were not exposed to much television, you might have followed a very disciplined sleep pattern of going to bed early and getting up early. You may be used to getting eight and one-half to nine hours of sleep each night.

The precise function of sleep is not yet fully understood. Most experts agree that sleep serves a primarily *restorative* function for the body. That is, during sleep we recover the physical and mental energy expelled during the day. This theory is supported by a great deal of research. For example, it is known that in children, the body grows more during sleep. Exercise and physical activity are known to affect sleep. Research has shown that people who get little exercise have lighter sleep than people who exercise regularly. However, it is not necessary to do strenuous exercise to make an impact on your sleep. Even mild forms of exercise and physical activity can result in experiencing more deep sleep. The benefits of physical activity on sleep will be discussed in more detail in chapter 14.

Deep sleep appears to be the most critical part of the sleep continuum as far as sleep's restorative properties are concerned. This is known from sleep deprivation studies in which volunteers over a number of nights are deprived of all or part of their sleep. On subsequent nights when they are allowed to sleep as much as they want, they spend more time in deep and REM sleep than usual. Because of this, it is felt that slow-wave and REM sleep are the most important stages of sleep. Another interesting finding from this research was that sleep deprived volunteers actually needed less sleep time overall on the recovery nights to get back their lost deep sleep. This is because they spent more time in deep sleep than they would have during a normal night's sleep. In one study, volunteers deprived of one night of sleep were able to recover their deep sleep after sleeping for only two hours. Volunteers deprived of two nights of sleep could recover their missed deep sleep in five hours.

Other research has shown that people who are short sleepers (that is, need only about six hours or less sleep every night) get nearly the same amount of deep sleep (and REM sleep) as normal sleepers. Hence, short sleepers seem to be more efficient sleepers, because they spend less time in the lighter sleep stages. However, short sleepers are not necessarily better sleepers because of this, rather they merely have learned how to "squeeze" the needed amount of restorative sleep out of a shorter sleep period.

The way we sleep seems to serve a purpose. It is generally thought that humans evolved to sleep at night to protect themselves from environmental dangers (predators, for example). Of course, there are different kinds of dangers at night in the modern world. The ever-busy, twenty-four-hour society in which we live has shortened the average length of time humans have available to sleep. One thing that has been preserved, however, is the sleep stage cycle. The fact that we reach waking states several times during the sleep period serves an important protective function. It would be undesirable to be in a deep sleep for eight hours straight. You would be unable to respond to an emergency such as a fire in the house or the cries of a sick child.

We know that sleep is very important for our lives. Sleep seems to serve primarily as a restorative mechanism for our bodies and minds. We need to sleep to "recharge our batteries." When we do not get enough sleep on one night, our bodies try to recover some of that sleep on the next night. Deep sleep shows the most recovery on such nights. For this reason, experts believe it is the most restful of all the sleep stages. The strategies in this book will show you how to get more deep sleep at night and ways to improve the efficiency of your sleep.

chapter 5

UTILIZING A SLEEP LOG

In this chapter you will learn:
- *How to record your nightly sleep*
- *The benefits of tracking your progress over the coming weeks*

An important part of the :60 Second program involves monitoring your progress via a daily sleep log. You will complete this :60 Second record every morning. On the form, you will record information about your previous night's sleep, such as how long it took you to fall asleep and the number of awakenings you had. Careful self-monitoring of your sleep is necessary so that you can assess the changes in your sleep that occur over the course of the program. It is important to start keeping the daily sleep log now.

With the sleep log you can document the pattern and severity of your sleep problems. You may be able to detect a specific pattern to your sleep problem, a continual series of which you were not previously aware. Part of the treatment can be focused on changing this pattern. Furthermore, the diary can actually be therapeutic. For example, some people find that after self-monitoring their sleep for a period, they discover that their sleep disturbances were not as severe as they originally believed and that they actually have several nights of good sleep in the course of the week. This helps reduce some of the anxiety they feel concerning their sleep problem.

:60 Second Daily Sleep Log

A copy of the sleep log follows. Additional copies are provided in Appendix C.

Step 1: The section below the title "To be completed in the evening" is to be done before you go to bed. Indicate your naps and the amounts of coffee, tea and cigarettes consumed each day.

Step 2: The remaining items on the sleep log should be completed in the morning, preferably upon rising, when your memory of the previous night is still fresh. People often find it difficult to remember exactly how long it took them to fall asleep or how many hours they slept, but give each of these items your best estimate.

Step 3: The sleep measures **Time in Bed (TIB)**, **Total Sleep Time (TST)** and **Sleep Efficiency (SEF)**, found at the bottom of the log form, are easily calculated from the information recorded on the sleep diary. Reminder: **Time in Bed** = Time went to bed (item #1) minus Time got out of bed (item #2). [Note: "Time got out of bed" may be different from the time when you woke up. For example, you may have awakened at 5:00 A.M., but stayed in bed for another two hours trying to get back to sleep until you finally got out of bed at 7:00 A.M. In this case, you would record 7:00 A.M. as the time you got out of bed, e.g., if you got into bed at 11:00 P.M. and got out of bed at 8:00 A.M., you would do the following calculation: 11:00 P.M.-8:00 A.M. = 9 hours spent in bed (Time in Bed).]

Total Sleep Time = estimated number of hours actually spent sleeping (item #3)

We can calculate the **Sleep Efficiency** ratio from the Time in Bed and Total Sleep Time figures.

Sleep Efficiency (%) = Total Sleep Time x 100 divided by Time in Bed.

This number represents the percentage of time you spend in bed actually sleeping. *Generally, as your sleep improves, your sleep efficiency ratio will increase.* The average sleep efficiency ratio for good sleepers is between 85 percent and 95 percent. A person with a sleep efficiency ratio above 90 percent is considered to have very good sleep. Someone with 100 percent sleep efficiency spends all of his or her time in bed asleep. There is space at the bottom of the sleep log to record your sleep efficiency ratio for each night. You can calculate this each night or wait until the end of the week to do all the nights at once.

Step 4: One common indicator of how well a person is sleeping is **Time to Fall Asleep** (item #4). The average time to fall asleep for healthy adults with no sleep problems is between ten and twenty minutes. However this value can range considerably.

Step 5: Another indicator that will be used to monitor your progress is the number of **Awakenings** you have during the night (item #5).

Step 6: Sleep efficiency and number of awakenings tell you how much sleep you are getting. They tell nothing about the **Quality** of your sleep; that is, whether you feel your sleep was refreshing and satisfying. In order to assess this aspect of your sleep, you are asked to make a rating of the quality of your sleep each morning. When making these ratings, it is important that you not compare yourself to someone without insomnia. Rather, you should judge each night's sleep on the basis of the best and worst night you have had since your sleep problem started. For example, if you feel your previous night's sleep was one of the best you have had in a long time, you should give it a rating of 4 or 5 on the scale. The same is true of the rating for how refreshing the previous night's sleep was for you.

Name: _____

SLEEP LOG for the week of _____ to _____

	SUN.	MON.	TUES.	WED.	THURS.	FRI.	SAT.
To be completed in the evening							
1. Did you take any naps today? (Y = Yes, N = No) If yes, give total length in minutes.							
2. How many cups of caffeinated coffee did you drink today?							
3. How many cups of caffeinated tea (i.e. not herbal) did you drink today?							
4. How many cigarettes did you smoke today?							
To be completed in the morning							
1. What time did you go to bed? (A.M./P.M.?)							
2. What time did you get out of bed? (A.M./P.M.?)							
3. Approximately how many hours of sleep did you get last night (to the nearest half hour)?							
4. How long did it take you to fall asleep?							
5. How many times did you wake up during the night?							
6. In the morning did you awaken at the time you wanted to? (E = Earlier, O = On time, L = Later)							
7. Rate the overall quality of your sleep (0 = Extremely Poor to 5 = Extremely Good)							
8. Rate how rested you felt this morning upon awakening (0 = Not at all Rested to 5 = Well Rested)							

$$\text{Sleep Efficiency} = \frac{\text{Total Sleep Time [\#3]}}{\text{Time Spent in Bed}} \times 100$$

Once you have a grasp of what the different items on the log are meant to measure, you should begin completing the Daily Sleep Log every morning from now until the end of the program. To understand what your sleep pattern is now, before treatment, fill out the log for two weeks before you attempt to make any changes to your sleep pattern.

:60 Second Progress Chart

We have included another form—the Sleep Diary (see below)—to record your weekly averages for the following sleep measures: Time to Fall Asleep, Sleep Efficiency, Number of Awakenings and Sleep Quality. We have also included four blank progress charts at the end of this chapter to help you keep track of your weekly progress on these measures. At the end of each week, you will total the daily figures for these four measures from the sleep log, divide by seven and write down that week's average for each of the four measures in the Sleep Diary. Then, you will take the weekly averages from the Sleep Diary and plot them on the respective progress charts. It is important that you keep track of making positive changes, so that you can follow your progress and try new things if you get stuck.

SLEEP DIARY

Diary Measure	WEEKLY AVERAGES FOR THE MONTH OF ____				
	1	2	3	4	5
Time to Fall Asleep					
Sleep Efficiency					
Awakenings					
Sleep Quality (#7 + #8)					

Diary Measure	WEEKLY AVERAGES FOR THE MONTH OF ____				
	6	7	8	9	10
Time to Fall Asleep					
Sleep Efficiency					
Awakenings					
Sleep Quality (#7 + #8)					

Sample Case: Doug's Sleep Diary

To ensure that you understand how to fill out your sleep log and plot your progress on the charts, let's walk through the steps of a sample case, based upon the sleep diaries of a person who went through this program. If you look at Doug's sleep log for his Baseline Week, you can see that he was having difficulty falling asleep and was spending a lot of time in bed awake. Let's work through the calculations for the first day of his sleep diary (Sunday).

Time in Bed = Time before midnight + Time after midnight
= 1.0 + 7.5

= 8.5 hours

Sleep Efficiency = Total Sleep Time x 100 ÷ by Time in Bed
= 4.5 x 100 / 8.5

= 52.9 (rounded to nearest whole number) = 53%

Doug also remembered that it took him a long time to fall asleep (about ninety minutes) and that he woke up a lot during the night (he could recall at least five different times). Overall, his sleep quality was not the worst he had experienced, but it was quite poor. He gave himself a rating of 2 on the scale for sleep quality and a 2 on the scale for feeling rested.

Doug kept careful records every morning for the whole week. Then at he end of the week, he calculated the average values for sleep efficiency, time to fall asleep, number of awakenings and sleep quality. He then entered these values on his progress charts.

For the next six weeks, as Doug completed the program, he kept filling out his sleep diary. Every week, he put his weekly averages onto his progress charts. Notice how the four charts on pages 48 and 49 clearly indicate marked improvement in Doug's sleep patterns. The charts gave Doug visual proof that his sleep was improving throughout the program and reinforced his desire to continue working to achieve normal sleep.

Keeping a similar record will help you on your path to a good night's rest.

Name: ___Doug___

SLEEP LOG for the week of March 1 to March 8

	SUN.	MON.	TUES.	WED.	THURS.	FRI.	SAT.
To be completed in the evening							
1. Did you take any naps today? (Y = Yes, N = No) If yes, give total length in minutes.	N	N	Y, 60 mins	N	Y, 30 mins	Y, 30 mins	N
2. How many cups of caffeinated coffee did you drink today?	2	3	5	4	6	1	5
3. How many cups of caffeinated tea (i.e. not herbal) did you drink today?	0	0	2	0	0	1	1
4. How many cigarettes did you smoke today?	12	15	20	25	20	18	16
To be completed in the morning							
1. What time did you go to bed? (A.M./P.M.?)	11:00	11:20	10:00	9:30	10:00	11:00	12:00
2. What time did you get out of bed? (A.M./P.M.?)	7:30	9:00	8:00	8:00	10:00	9:30	8:30
3. Approximately how many hours of sleep did you get last night (to the nearest half hour)?	4.5	6	5.5	7	8	5.5	6.5
4. How long did it take you to fall asleep?	90	25	60	90	35	40	45
5. How many times did you wake up during the night?	5	2	1	4	4	3	2
6. In the morning did you awaken at the time you wanted to? (E = Earlier, O = On time, L = Later)	E	O	L	E	E	E	L
7. Rate the overall quality of your sleep (0 = Extremely Poor to 5 = Extremely Good)	2	3	3	1	2	3	2
8. Rate how rested you felt this morning upon awakening (0 = Not at all Rested to 5 = Well Rested)	2	2	4	0	3	3	2
Sleep Efficiency = Total Sleep Time [#3] X 100 / Time Spent in Bed	53%	62%	55%	66%	66%	52%	76%

Doug's Progress Charts

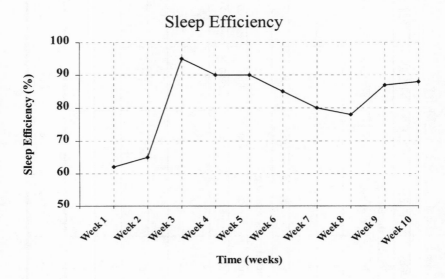

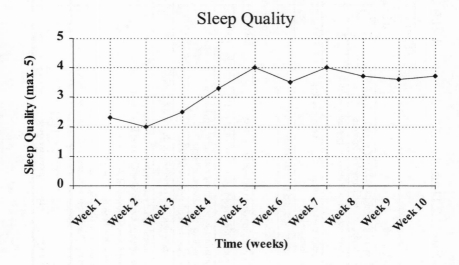

Doug's Progress Charts

Time to Fall Asleep

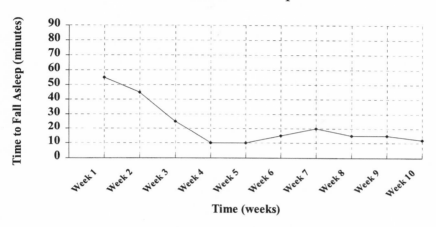

Number of Awakenings

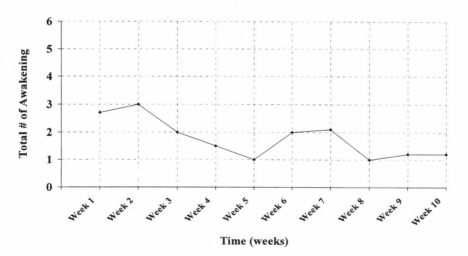

My Progress Charts

Sleep Efficiency

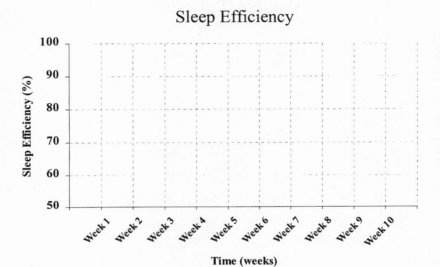

Sleep Quality

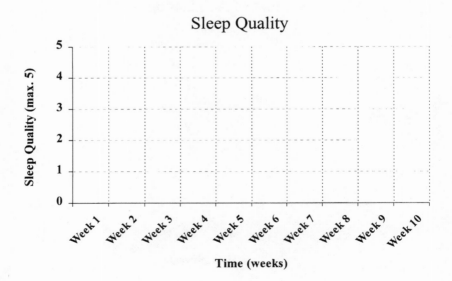

My Progress Charts

Time to Fall Asleep

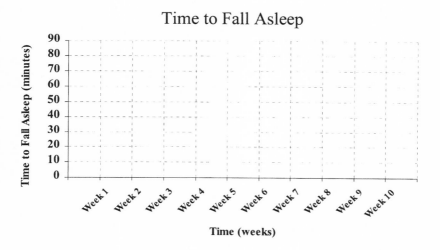

Number of Awakenings

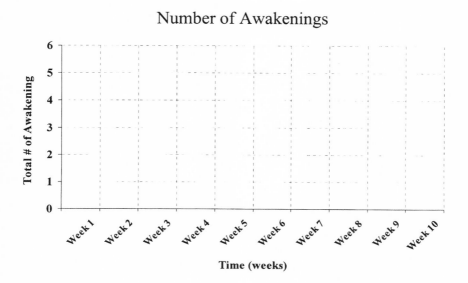

PART 2

:60 SECOND BEHAVIOR CHANGE TECHNIQUES

chapter **6**

SLEEP MORE, WORRY LESS: RESTRICTING YOUR TIME IN BED

In this chapter you will:

- *Learn why staying in bed is not always the best way to cope with a sleep problem*
- *Start the sleep restriction method to concentrate your sleep period and get more deep sleep*

Review Daily Sleep Log

Before proceeding with the :60 Second behavior change techniques, review your daily sleep log records and progress charts for the previous two weeks. You may have started to notice things about your sleep of which you were not previously aware. For example, do your sleep problems persist through the entire week or do you actually experience a number of good nights? Do your bad nights tend to cluster together around the same time of the week—weekends for example? Do you sleep better when you don't nap during the day?

Focus on your good nights now. Did you do anything different on those days as compared with the days when you had your bad nights? Were you more active on your good days, for example? Did you smoke less or consume less coffee? Try to identify behaviors that may be having an influence on your sleep. Finding such behaviors is an important step to realizing that your sleep problems now are at least partially under your control. Recognizing that some sleep problems are the results of your own daytime actions means that you can do something about them. By changing or modifying your behaviors you can improve your quality of sleep.

Behavior Change Techniques

Here are some specific techniques you can use to make your sleep better. Keep in mind, we will be discussing a number of different strategies for coping with sleep disturbances, some of which will work well for some people and some of which will work well for others. Don't get discouraged if you try a particular technique and find you do not meet with complete success. Instead, go on to the next. It is important to try all of them so that you can figure out which ones work best for you and how and when to combine them. Eventually you will find combinations of techniques that are effective in most situations.

As mentioned in chapter 3, it is common for people with insomnia to develop several bad sleep habits. Here is a checklist of behaviors which may negatively influence your sleep.

:60 Second Behavior Checklist

_____ Get up or go to bed at different times every day
_____ Nap during the day
_____ Spend a lot of time in bed at night not sleeping
_____ Use the bed to relax or rest—but not sleep—during the day
_____ Use the bed or bedroom for activities other than sleep or sex (e.g., watch television, read, eat)
_____ Lie in bed at night worrying about the day's events or your sleep problems

If you have checked any of these items, you may be contributing to your sleep problems. Most people engage in these activities as a means of coping with sleep loss. For example, if you have a bad night you may feel it necessary to nap the next day to cope with the fatigue. However, research indicates that in the long run this habit only serves to perpetuate sleep problems. You can see how easy it is for a vicious cycle of bad sleep habits and poor sleep to develop.

The objective of this section of the book is to limit these and other problematic sleep connected activities as much as possible. By doing this, you will break the vicious cycle. This is a well-established technique to short-circuit the poor sleep cycle and stabilize your sleep pattern.

In this chapter and the next, you will be introduced to the following coping strategies for attaining better sleep:
1. Sleep restriction
2. Stimulus control

Remember that these techniques have been well-researched and found to be effective with people suffering from chronic sleep problems. These techniques may not cure your sleep problems, but they will correct some of the factors that may be maintaining your insomnia. We'll start with the sleep restriction method.

:60 Second Sleep Restriction Method

Do you notice how the longer you spend in bed, the worse your sleep seems? The goal of the sleep restriction method is to gradually concentrate your sleep into a shorter period of time spent in bed. This will be accomplished by getting you to limit the amount of time you spend in bed and bringing it closer to the amount of time you actually spend asleep. With this method you will become a more efficient sleeper.

The thinking behind this procedure is based on the fact that many people with insomnia spend too much time in bed at night not sleeping. If you can only sleep five and one-half hours a night, then spending eight hours in bed is only making your sleep problems worse. Those extra hours are probably being spent feeling frustrated and becoming progressively more anxious and upset, rather than sleeping. Your body eventually comes to recognize that your bed is a place where you *stay awake* rather than get to sleep.

Try the following. Review your daily sleep log records for the past two weeks. Find two or more occasions when your time spent sleeping was similar, but your time in bed was very different. Your sleep efficiency ratio probably was higher on the nights you spent less time in bed. Now check your ratings for sleep quality and feeling refreshed on those nights. Did you rate your sleep quality as higher on the nights you spent less time in bed? Even if your sleep quality was the same, you have just made an important realization: **Spending more time in bed doesn't make you sleep better.** Most people with insomnia try to cope with their inability to get enough sleep by spending more time in bed in hopes of recovering lost sleep. They frequently go to bed early, hoping to catch up on sleep loss with extra hours in bed. Ironically, this is the worst thing you can do since it only strengthens the negative association of lying awake in bed. Even if you do recover some sleep, it will be fragmented, light and ultimately unsatisfying. Research has shown that a shorter period of continuous, uninterrupted sleep is more refreshing than the same amount of poor quality sleep spread over a longer period. Think of what you could accomplish with those hours spent in bed but not sleeping!

Before beginning this procedure, you should have a good understanding of the sleep measures **time in bed, total sleep time** and **sleep efficiency.** You should know how to calculate each of these measures for your own sleep. If you don't, go back to chapter 5 and review the material on these measures. Here are the step-by-step instructions for applying sleep restriction:

Step 1: Look at your sleep log and calculate your average sleep efficiency for the past week. (i.e., add the sleep efficiency values for the past seven days and divide by seven; the average should be a value that makes sense—if it is out of proportion, greater than 100 percent for example, you have made an error in calculation). This value is your current, overall sleep efficiency. The object of the sleep restriction procedure will be to increase this value to your target goal value (e.g., greater than 85 percent sleep efficiency).

Note: If you calculate your average sleep efficiency to be greater than 90 percent, your sleep efficiency is good and you don't have to continue with this procedure.

Step 2: From your sleep log, calculate your average nightly total sleep time (TST). This will be your "sleep window" (i.e., amount of time from bedtime to arising).

Step 3: Starting tonight, restrict the amount of time you spend in bed (TIB) to the value for your sleep window. It is best to do this by going to bed later at night rather than getting up earlier in the morning. When you are trying to improve your sleep, you should try to maintain a regular arising time each morning.

Note: Never go below five hours for your sleep window; if your average nightly total sleep time is less than this amount, then use five hours as your starting sleep window.

Step 4: After one week of 100 percent or nearly 100 percent sleep efficiency, increase the amount of time you spend in bed by fifteen minute intervals every week until your sleep efficiency is near or higher than 85 percent. Continue to complete your sleep log. Don't add fifteen minutes until you have followed the sleep restriction guidelines for one or two weeks and you have begun to notice some improvements (e.g., fewer awakenings, reduced time to fall asleep). Stop adding fifteen minutes to your sleep window when your sleep efficiency stabilizes at 85 percent or higher for at least one week. A worksheet is provided to help you with this method.

Step 5: It is important that you do not nap during the day. You may feel like you are not getting enough sleep during the first week of this procedure, but you should not try to compensate by napping. This will interfere with the sleep restriction process. However, use common sense with this guideline. If you need to drive for a long period or you are going to operate dangerous equipment, by all means take a nap if you are feeling too tired to work safely.

:60 Second Sleep Restriction Worksheet

Determine your sleep window:
What was the average number of hours you spent sleeping each night for the past seven days?
_____hours. This is your **sleep window.**

Week 1	time in bed = _____ (sleep window)*	} sleep efficiency = __100%__
	total sleep time = _____	
Week 2	time in bed = _____ (sleep window + 15 mins)	} sleep efficiency = _____
	total sleep time = _____	
Week 3	time in bed = _____ (sleep window + 30 mins)	} sleep efficiency = _____
	total sleep time = _____	

In the remaining weeks, you can continue to add time in bed as long as your sleep efficiency is above 85 percent.

Week 4	time in bed = _____	} sleep efficiency = _____
	total sleep time = _____	
Week 5	time in bed = _____	} sleep efficiency = _____
	total sleep time = _____	
Week 6	time in bed = _____	} sleep efficiency = _____
	total sleep time = _____	
Week 7	time in bed = _____	} sleep efficiency = _____
	total sleep time = _____	

* For the first week, your time in bed will be equal to your sleep window, making your sleep efficiency ratio 100 percent.

How Does Sleep Restriction Work?

One of the reasons why this procedure works well is that it actually concentrates your sleep into a shorter time period spent in bed, giving you more refreshing deep sleep. Although you are sleeping about the same amount of time, your sleep will be more efficient, less fragmented and ultimately more refreshing. More of your sleep period will be spent in deep sleep. When you get up in the morning and recall the night's sleep, you will remember sleeping most of the time while in bed. You won't remember that long, frustrating period when you lay in bed trying to get to sleep, because it did not occur.

To illustrate the benefits of having "concentrated" sleep, consider the following. Have you ever had a really refreshing short nap? A time when you were very tired, lay down for an hour and slept the whole hour? You probably woke up feeling a little tired, but generally feeling refreshed. This would constitute a "concentrated" sleep session. It probably didn't take you long to fall asleep and you probably didn't wake up much. Many naps are like a mini night's sleep, but usually more concentrated in deep sleep. Ideally you would like your nighttime sleep to resemble this "concentrated" short nap (except longer of course!). The advantages and disadvantages of naps will be discussed later in more detail.

Another reason why sleep restriction works is that, initially, you are subjecting your body to a state of sleep deprivation. Sleeping in a state of deprivation allows you to fall asleep sooner, have fewer awakenings and spend more time in deep sleep. You will remember from chapter 4 how volunteers deprived of sleep spend more time in deep sleep. When you shorten your sleep period your body still retains the same amount of deep sleep. You wake up from a more concentrated period of deep sleep. Of course, this will only occur if you keep from napping during the day. Having a nap will rob you of your night's deep sleep.

Sleep restriction works even better when combined with other personal coping strategies and techniques. Sleep restriction and the guidelines in the next chapter, for example, compliment each other and should be practiced together. We will discuss stimulus control procedures in the next chapter.

:60 Second Tips for Success with Sleep Restriction

1. Use the steps as guidelines, but use your own judgment as to how much you increase your time in bed each week (for example, fifteen, thirty or forty-five minutes). Don't use increments of less than fifteen minutes since it will be too difficult to monitor your progress.
2. Don't reduce your time in bed to anything less than five hours no matter how poor your sleep efficiency is. If you are only sleeping two to three hours per night in total, you should try some of the other procedures in this book first to increase your total sleep time.
3. Avoid altering your arising time in the morning. Decrease your time in bed by going to bed later. If you are now in the habit of arising at 6:00 A.M. every morning, stick to that. You may find, however, that applying sleep restriction will force you to alter your regular arising time. For example, if you are in the habit of waking up at 4:00 A.M. and lying in bed until 6:00 A.M. before arising, then by all means get out of bed earlier. Use 4:00 A.M. as your arising time if you absolutely must.
4. Initially, your sleep may seem worse or it may seem as though you are fighting sleepiness in order to comply with your sleep window. Don't let this discourage you. Keep in mind that it takes at least two weeks for you to adjust to the new sleep schedule. A little short-term discomfort now is a small price to pay for long-term satisfaction.
5. Another common reaction to sleep restriction during the first couple of weeks in the program is feeling sleepy during the day. Nevertheless, avoid daytime napping. This will disrupt the sleep rhythm you are trying to develop with this technique and lessen its benefits.
6. If you find the sleep restriction procedures too complicated to apply, you can use the simpler "rule-of-thumb" approach:

Abbreviated Sleep Restriction Method

In general, your time in bed should never exceed your total sleeping time by more than **one hour** (this includes the time it takes you to fall asleep, awakenings and time spent in bed after awakening in the morning). For example, if you are sleeping an average of five hours per night, then you should not be spending more than six hours lying in bed.

chapter 7

CHANGING SLEEP HABITS FOR THE BETTER

In this chapter you will:
*   *Review your progress using sleep restriction procedures*
*   *Learn a set of techniques designed to build a positive association between your bed and sleeping—stimulus control*

Progress with Sleep Restriction

You should be into your second week of sleep restriction. Many people find this a difficult period. You may find it hard to stick to the sleep restriction rules. You may feel sleepier during the day than before you started. These are all natural reactions to using the sleep restriction techniques. Changing old habits is tough. However, a little discomfort now is a small hardship for longlasting improvement in your sleep. Review your progress on a weekly basis and don't worry about whether the difficulties will last forever, because they won't.

As an incentive, take a look at your progress chart for the past week. Your sleep efficiency should be at or very close to 100 percent for every night during the first week you started sleep restriction. Your time to fall asleep will probably shorten for most nights as well since you are probably falling asleep soon after you allow yourself to go to bed. The daytime sleepiness you may be experiencing will gradually go away as you start to increase your time in bed and set a routine. The next procedures will help you stick with sleep restriction.

Stimulus Control Procedures

This chapter has one primary objective: to help you re-establish and strengthen the association between sleeping and your bed. Many of the habits people with insomnia develop are incompatible with maintaining regular and satisfying sleep routines. We reviewed some of these at the beginning of the last chapter (napping in the afternoon, spending waking hours in bed doing other activities, etc.). For people with chronic sleep problems, the bed and bedroom often become associated with activities other than sleeping. To help break this association, psychologist Dr. Richard Bootzin developed a set of strategies or "rules" for insomniacs to follow. These strategies are collectively referred to as stimulus control procedures. Stimulus control is a behavior change technique that helps people break negative associations (like between your bed and restlessness) and build healthier associations. Stimulus control has also been used to help people quit smoking and lose weight. The goal of stimulus control for sleep is to get you to phase out habits or routines that are interfering with your sleep pattern. Since this may be difficult to do at first, we will provide you with important tips to help you achieve your goal.

:60 Second Sleep Habit Modification

Unlike sleep restriction techniques, the application of stimulus control is not guided by a formula. Rather, it is a set of guidelines and instructions on how to break certain habits working against good sleep, while at the same time reinforcing other sleep-friendly behaviors. The primary goal is to reestablish and strengthen the association between your bed and sleeping. The list which follows summarizes the stimulus control procedures.

:60 Second Stimulus Control Techniques

Do not use your bed or bedroom for anything other than sleep and sex.
Why? To build up the association between your bedroom and sleeping.

Establish a set of regular bedtime routines to signal the approach of bedtime. Do these activities in the same order every night.

Allow yourself at least an hour before bedtime to unwind.
Why? To establish a pattern to make every day seem more the same. Make going to bed a habit. Eventually, you will associate your presleep routine with feeling sleepy.

Go to bed only when you are sleepy.
Why? To stop trying to sleep when you are not tired. Going to bed when you are not sleepy only prolongs the time you will spend in bed trying to get to sleep.

When you get into bed, turn out the lights with the intention of going right to sleep. If you cannot fall asleep within a reasonable time (about twenty minutes), get up and go into another room; engage in some quiet, non-stimulating activity until you begin to feel ready to sleep, then get back into bed.
Why? To break the vicious cycle of trying to get to sleep with no success. The frustration and anxiety over not getting to sleep leads you to be ever more aroused, making sleep even less likely. Breaking the cycle will reduce this frustration and make sleep come easier.

If you still do not fall asleep within a brief time, repeat the previous step. Repeat this process as often as it is necessary throughout the night. Use this same procedure if you awaken in the middle of the night and do not return to sleep within about twenty minutes.
Why? Same as above.

Get up at the same time in the morning regardless of how much you slept.
Why? To establish a strong, regular sleep and waking schedule.

Avoid daytime napping, especially after 3:00 P.M.
Why? To reserve your sleep for nighttime only. Sleeping in the afternoon is like starting your nighttime sleep period early; doing so will result in your nighttime sleep being shorter and more fragmented.

Let's go through these techniques in greater detail one at a time.

1. Do not use the bed or bedroom for any activity other than sleep and sex. The reason for this rule is to get you to associate your bedroom with sleeping and little else. This means you should not watch television, eat or do anything else in your sleeping space. Reading is okay, as long as you do it before sleep (don't read in bed during the day) and choose pleasurable reading materials. Adhering to this rule will help you to break the negative association between your bed and not sleeping and reduce the feelings of frustration, anxiety and helplessness that may have plagued you. Your goal is to make your bed sleep-friendly.

   Tips: Another way to look at this rule is to think in terms of developing positive sleep habits. Most of the habits people have are formed by a strong association between a specific environment and a set of behaviors. For example, have you ever walked into the kitchen and suddenly felt hungry? The feeling gets even stronger when you open the refrigerator door! What is your response to this feeling? You probably make yourself something to eat. This is because going to the kitchen and getting something to eat is a habit for most people. Being in the kitchen environment brings on feelings of hunger and serves as the cue or stimulus for a set of behaviors to occur.

   Think of this example as a model for what you want to achieve with the stimulus control procedure. For people who sleep well, their bed acts as a cue to feel sleepy and fall asleep quickly (think of those people who tell you that they fall asleep as soon as their heads hit their pillows). Your goal should be to see if you can reach the point where you walk into your bedroom and feel sleepy. The way to do this is to not do anything else in your bedroom other than sleep. Obviously, this becomes somewhat difficult if you live in a one-room apartment. In this case, you will have to use your imagination and ingenuity to come up with some alternatives. Here are some suggestions, however:

1) Concentrate your bedroom furniture to one corner or space in the room and don't use that area except at night when you want to go to sleep.
2) If you use your bed to read or watch television, STOP! Turn the television away from the bed. Investing in a comfortable

reading chair will be money well spent if it results in your sleeping better in the long-run.

3) Get a divider, perhaps a decorative screen, to physically separate your bed from the rest of the room.

4) Trade in your bed for a fold-up futon that can also be used as a couch. When the futon is unfolded to become a bed, that will be your cue to feel sleepy.

2. Establish a bedtime routine to signal the onset of sleep. Your goal with this procedure is to develop a ritual set of behaviors that for you clearly *separates day and night.* Thus, reserve a set of activities to do only before going to bed. Perform these activities every night until they become a routine. This will be your presleep ritual. Ensure that none of the activities in your presleep ritual is contrary to inducing sleep. Examples of such counter-sleep activities are: (a) having a cup of coffee or regular tea; (b) reading stressful or stimulating material; (c) exercising. Some examples of productive pre-sleep activities are: (a) taking a warm bath; (b) laying out clothes to wear for the next day (or any other activity which makes it easier for you to get up in the morning); (c) practicing relaxation techniques (to be discussed in more detail in the next chapter); (d) having a light snack or cup of herbal tea; and (e) reading an enjoyable, light novel.

Tips: Ideally, your presleep routine should consist of mostly sleep-friendly or neutral activities. If your routine consists mostly of neutral behaviors, consider incorporating a few relaxing activities. This can be something as simple as reading a good book or taking a bath. Try to make the one-hour period before going to bed a time to wind down. In other words, consider activities that will clear any anxious thoughts out of your mind and will gradually put your body into a state of relaxation.

3. Go to bed only when you are sleepy. There is no reason to go to bed if you are not tired enough to fall asleep. Getting into bed prematurely will only prolong the time you spend lying in bed awake, becoming frustrated and tense. Going to bed early only gives you more time to conjure up unpleasant memories of the day behind you, worry about tomorrow's events and ruminate over your sleep problem. All of these strengthen the association between your bedroom and not sleeping when your goal should be the exact opposite.

Tips: This strategy goes hand in hand with the sleep restriction method in which you delay your time going to bed. Make sure bedtime is late enough to ensure you fall asleep soon after going to bed. If you don't get to sleep quickly, the next strategy will help you.

4. Get out of bed if you can't fall asleep within a reasonable time period. What is a reasonable time period? Some sleep specialists will say ten to fifteen minutes is long enough to wait. Others will say twenty to thirty minutes. The fact is that it depends on the individual and what is reasonable for you. Never wait more than thirty minutes before making the decision to get out of bed.

Tips: It is important that you do not watch the clock every few minutes when applying this rule, for such behavior will only draw your attention to your sleeplessness, causing you to be more stimulated. You should be able to estimate in your mind when your personal time criterion has elapsed. If you find yourself watching the clock, then this is probably a sign that you are not yet tired enough to sleep and ought not to be in bed yet.

When you get out of bed, leave your bedroom altogether to remove yourself from all associations of sleeplessness. Engage in some non-stimulating activity while you wait to become sleepy. Here are a few suggestions:

Non-stimulating Pursuits for the Sleepless
- Listen to relaxing music
- Take a hot bath
- Organize a stack of coupons
- Watch a boring movie
- Read a boring book
- Sort through your recycling box

Do not lie down on the couch. Many people find that they can't get to sleep in their bed, but when they lie down on the couch they can fall asleep within ten minutes. What does this mean? Likely, their bed and bedroom have become associated with the inability to sleep. The couch, on the other hand, starting out as a neutral object, has now become associated with sleeping. You may argue that since getting to sleep is the goal, sleeping on the couch should be all right. Unfortunately, doing this repeatedly will only reinforce the sleep-inhibiting quality of your bedroom and turn your otherwise neutral couch into a positive sleep-promoting zone. Unless you want to spend the rest of your life sleeping on the couch at night, it's probably best to avoid this activity as much as possible.

5. Repeat the procedure throughout the night every time you can't get to sleep within a reasonable time period. This is one of the most difficult rules to follow. Admittedly, getting out of your warm, comfortable bed is hard to do at 3:00 A.M. However, just remember that there's no point lying in bed if you are not sleeping and it will be counterproductive in the end.

   Tips: To make it easier to get out of bed, try the following tricks: (a) Leave a warm bathrobe and pair of slippers at the foot of your bed so that exposing yourself to the cold room air will not be a deterrent to getting up; (b) Plan to have your non-stimulating activities ready and available (for example, put a videotape in the VCR, book on the table, etc.); (c) Avoid clock-watching to prevent becoming anxious or distressed at the thought of having to get up at an irregular hour.

   When you get out of bed, make sure you don't return until a reasonable time has elapsed. As a rule of thumb, stay out of bed for at least twenty-five minutes. Try to follow this procedure even if you think you can fall asleep before twenty-five minutes have elapsed. Don't confuse feeling fatigued with feeling sleepy. Getting out of bed at 3:00 A.M. may leave you feeling sluggish, but this doesn't always translate into the ability to sleep. Also remember that the longer you stay up and prolong sleep, the faster sleep will come when you do get back into bed.

6. Get up at the same time every morning. Set your alarm clock for a specific hour and get out of bed when it goes off. Do this regardless of how much or little you slept and on both weekdays and weekends.

Research indicates that all animals, including humans, have an internal biological clock that regulates how much time we should spend sleeping and how much time we should spend awake for every twenty-four hour period. This internal sleep-wake schedule is also called a circadian rhythm ("circadian" is Latin for 'about a day'). The sleep-wake circadian rhythm is actually linked to other internal biological rhythms. Body temperature, for example, fluctuates during the twenty-four hour day, with the lowest value occurring in the early morning when most people are still sleeping.

Circadian rhythms take some time to develop, but once they do they are a powerful force in our need to sleep. When the individual tries to compensate for a poor night's sleep with bed rest and napping, the sleep rhythm is disrupted. To help your circadian sleep rhythm return to or arrive at a more regular cycle, it is important to minimize the number of disruptions. Maintaining a regular rising time is one important step towards doing this. Another way to think of this strategy is to imagine that a regular wake-up time is an anchor on to which your otherwise irregular sleep rhythm can hold.

Tips: This can be a challenging rule to follow if you don't have regulated daytime activities. However, following this daily rising time becomes even more important, because the temptation to stay in bed is greater when you have no job or other activity which demands a regular starting time. To overcome the temptation of staying late in bed, particularly if you've experienced poor sleep, you might consider planning a regular activity every morning so that you must get up at a scheduled time. For example, plan your daily stretching exercises or a morning walk for first thing after you get out of bed. If you do any volunteer work or other out of home activity, arrange to do it in the morning. These are just suggestions; your own schedule and personal interests will determine how you may wish to handle maintaining a sleep/rise schedule.

7. Avoid daytime napping. The longer you stay awake during the day, the easier sleep should come at night. Studies have shown that the amount of time people spend awake during the day can predict how long it will take them to fall asleep and how long they will stay asleep. For example, someone who is active for fifteen hours of the day will take less time to fall asleep at night than if they were awake for only ten hours.

In addition to prolonging the onset of sleep, a nap can also rob your night's sleep of precious, restorative deep sleep. When you nap, especially in the afternoon, your sleep resembles the first part of the sleep cycle that is highly concentrated in deep sleep. Your body only needs so much deep sleep in a twenty-four hour period and using it up in an afternoon nap means less deep sleep at night.

If you must nap, consider doing it in the morning. A morning nap is more of a continuation of the previous night's sleep and is therefore less likely to interfere with the coming night. Having an afternoon nap is like starting your sleep period early and only serves to fragment your night's sleep.

Tips: Avoiding daytime napping is a hard procedure to follow. Many people find that as the day wears on, their fatigue increases with activity. This makes taking a nap in the afternoon seem necessary. Strategies, such as pacing (that is, spreading out your activities into manageable chunks), can be used to prevent a build-up of fatigue caused by doing too much activity at once. Another strategy is to find alternative activities to napping. When you feel the urge to nap, go for a walk. Always choose an activity that takes you out of the house. Being in the house close to your bedroom or the couch may be too great a temptation.

As mentioned previously, the napping rule should be applied with a little common sense. For example, you should never drive a motor vehicle or operate hazardous, heavy equipment if you are feeling tired; in such cases, by all means take a nap! Remember that an occasional nap is not necessarily harmful. However, regular napping will be counterproductive to your progress in the :60 Second sleep-ease program.

:60 Second Tips for Success Applying Stimulus Control Procedures

1. Copy the seven strategies and display them in a visible place (e.g., on your refrigerator door) to serve as a reminder.
2. Follow most of the rules. Especially important are the rules about getting and staying out of bed when you can't sleep after a reasonable time period. These rules are the heart of stimulus control.

3. Don't confuse feeling fatigued with feeling sleepy when trying to gauge if you are ready to go to bed. Remember that sleep is controlled by the mind, not the body.

4. Choose non-stimulating activities that can be finished easily or stopped after twenty-five minutes when you can't sleep. For example, read a short story, magazine or do a crossword puzzle. Avoid engaging in activities like playing computer/video games or watching a suspenseful movie.

5. Enlist the help and support of your spouse or roommate. Show them the list of guidelines so that they are aware of what you are doing. Some people feel guilty about getting out of bed when they can't sleep for fear of waking up their sleeping partner. To alleviate such feelings, make sure your partner is aware of your program to stop insomnia. Your partner probably finds your tossing and turning to be more disruptive than you simply getting in and out of bed once or twice.

6. Avoid clock-watching. Set your alarm for your regular wake-up time, but turn the face of the clock away from your bed.

7. Adjust your pre-bedtime routine to coincide with your practice of sleep restriction. That is, start your pre-bedtime routine in the one-hour period prior to your new bedtime according to the sleep restriction schedule you are on.

8. Schedule some pleasurable activities in the evening. Try to break the monotony of watching television after dinner and waiting for your bedtime. Simply passing time until it is time to go to bed just gives you more opportunity to worry about your sleep. Find activities to do that take you out of your house or apartment. More suggestions are:
   - Go to a movie on a night you don't normally go
   - Take in a concert or evening sports event
   - Go for a walk with your spouse or a friend
   - Arrange a night with friends to play cards
   - Eat out in a restaurant

chapter **8**

EVALUATING SLEEP MEDICATIONS

In this chapter you will:
* *Learn about sleep medications, how they work and how they affect your sleep*
* *Find out the right way to reduce sleep medications*

The purpose of this section is to inform you about the effects of sleep altering medications and some of the risks involved in taking them on a long-term basis. Most of the information in this section will focus on the hypnotics (sleeping pills). However, some discussion will also be devoted to the other medications that affect sleep. How to reduce or eliminate sleep medications will be discussed and specific guidelines for medication withdrawal will be provided.

Benzodiazepine Medications

Most sleeping pills prescribed today belong to a class of drugs called the benzodiazepines. Older sleeping pills such as barbiturates and chloral hydrate are rarely used anymore, because they tend to have more side effects and are generally not very safe to take for long periods. Benzodiazepine medications are very popular sleeping pills. In 1993, over eighteen million prescriptions for benzodiazepines were written in the United States alone and millions more worldwide. All sleep medications have trade names (given by the pharmaceutical companies that market the drugs) and generic names (abbreviated forms of the long chemical name). For example, the drug temazepam

goes by the trade name of Restoril. Commonly prescribed benzodiazepines are flurazepam (Dalmane), nitrazepam (Mogadon) and tria-
zolam (Halcion). All these medications have similar effects in the
brain of the users. They differ however in their duration of action.
For example, there are short, medium and long-acting sleeping pills.
Medications that are short-acting are mostly broken down by the
body before waking. In contrast, the active chemicals in long-acting
sleeping pills such as Dalmane accumulate with repeated usage. The
metabolites (the chemicals that remain when a drug is broken down
by the liver) of long-acting benzodiazepines are actually more benzodiazepines! It is almost like taking several drugs at once. Long-acting
medications often lead to waking up feeling drowsy and confused.
One benefit of a shorter-acting sleeping pill is that such "hangover"
effects are greatly reduced. The downside is that short-acting sleeping
pills don't always help with awakenings later in the night. A long-acting pill will probably keep you sleeping until morning, but at the
expense of waking up with a hungover feeling. The medium-acting
medication Restoril is considered an all-purpose drug because its
duration of action is sufficient to cover an entire sleep period with
fewer side effects in the morning.

Non-benzodiazepine Medications
There are newer drugs on the market that are technically not benzodiazepines but have similar actions in the brain. One of these is zopiclone (Imovane), which is not available in the United States, but is
widely marketed in Canada and Europe. Zopiclone seems to have
fewer side effects and, thus, may be better for regular use. This medication is medium-acting and does not seem to have the same detrimental effects on deep sleep stages (this is discussed more in the section "How do sleeping pills work?"). Nevertheless, most physicians
are cautious in prescribing zopiclone for long-term use because the
possibility of addiction may be just as likely as with use of benzodiazepines. Two other non-benzodiazepine drugs are zolpiden (Ambien)
and zaleplon (Starnoc). Both of these drugs are available in the United
States and Europe. Zaleplon is an ultra short-acting drug. It can get
you to sleep quickly, but does not help with mid-sleep awakenings.

New and improved sleep medications often promise better sleep and fewer side effects. This can be tempting to someone with chronic insomnia. However, be aware that many "new" medications are often not that new. Pharmaceutical companies can only keep the medications they develop patent-protected for a limited number of years before other companies are legally allowed to make generic versions. A "new" drug is sometimes an old drug with a minor variation in its chemical structure that is being sold at a higher price.

Other Medications That Affect Sleep

Tricyclic antidepressants are frequently prescribed for their sleep enhancing properties. Common tricyclic antidepressants include amitriptyline (Elavil), doxepin (Sinequan), empramine (Tofranil) and clomipramine (Anafranil). Other medications that seem to help people sleep better are trazodone (Desyrel) and nefazodone (Serzone). These medications need to be taken at bedtime to help with the problem of insomnia. The most common side effects of the tricyclic antidepressants include dry mouth, daytime drowsiness and weight gain. Rarer side effects include hypotension (low blood pressure), blurred vision, constipation and nightmares. Overall, the side effects seem to be better tolerated by most persons, making the tricyclic antidepressants safer for regular use than the benzodiazepines. Even so, many people find that when their confidence increases as a result of using self-management approaches to handle their sleep problems, they can gradually wean themselves off all medications.

There are numerous over-the-counter medications that you can get without a prescription. Most of these are antihistamines that cause mild drowsiness. They are usually not very effective for persons with severe, chronic insomnia. In fact, they can be dangerous because some people take larger than recommended doses in order to achieve sleep.

Many medications that are taken for other reasons can worsen insomnia. The class of antidepressants known as SSRI's (selective-serotonin receptive inhibitors) can have a stimulating effect, keeping you awake. Examples of SSRI's are Prozac, Paxil, Wellbutrin and Zoloft. Approximately 5 to 20 percent of individuals taking SSRI's for depression will develop insomnia. Generally, the higher the dosage, the greater the chances of sleep problems developing. This side effect may lessen over time and should resolve itself completely when the drug is discontinued.

How Do Sleeping Pills Work?

Hypnotic drugs are in the same class as the anti-anxiety medications, such as diazepam (Valium), alprazolam (Xanax) and lorazepam (Ativan). Therefore, one of the ways in which sleeping pills seem to work is to reduce the anxiety of not being able to get to sleep. In some ways, insomnia has a lot in common with anxiety. The stress of worrying about whether or not you will get to sleep causes arousal and keeps you awake. We know that having a relaxed mind is an important condition for getting to sleep. Taking a sleeping pill is a quick but artificial way of achieving a state of mental relaxation.

Of course, sleeping pills do more than just reduce anxiety. They also cause extreme drowsiness that helps you fall asleep and stay in a state of sleep for several hours. Most people find that the length of their sleep increases with sleeping pills. However, the sleep that you do get is not normal. Most sleeping pills increase the amount of light sleep (stages 1 and 2), while decreasing the amount of deep sleep and REM sleep. You may sleep more, but at the expense of your deep sleep, which is the most restorative stage of sleep for your body. Along with a groggy "hangover" feeling, you may still feel tired the next day. The tiredness is your body's way of saying it didn't get enough deep sleep. In addition, hypnotic drugs can cause memory problems and liver damage if taken at high doses for long periods of time.

Tryptophan

"Drink a glass of warm milk to help you sleep." Sound familiar? Well, this old wives' tale may have some scientific basis. Milk contains the amino acid tryptophan which is a chemical the brain needs in order to manufacture another chemical, serotonin. This latter chemical is a neurotransmitter that helps the body slow down and go to sleep. Tryptophan is also found in many foods like fish, eggs and poultry. So all you have to do is drink milk, eat these foods and your sleep will improve, right? Actually, it is not that simple. One of the problems is that the amount of tryptophan in these sources is so small that you would have to eat dozens of eggs or gallons of milk to get enough extra tryptophan in your body to make a substantial difference. This, of course, is not very practical and certainly not very healthy.

Tryptophan (or l-tryptophan on some labels) has been available in a pure tablet form for many years. Some doctors will prescribe tryptophan in dosages of two to six grams as a sleep aid. It is also used to help some antidepressant medications work better. The research on tryptophan's effectiveness as a sleep aid has produced mixed results. Some studies say that it helps, others say it does very little for sleep. Many studies have been conducted on people with mild insomnia and some have used student volunteers with normal sleep. It is hard to know if tryptophan helps when the research subject's sleep was almost normal in the first place. People who take tryptophan for sleep need to take a dose every night for several weeks for the drug to have any chance of working. Taking the pill once in a while will not have much effect on your sleep.

The side effects of tryptophan are minimal. A blood disorder called eosinophiliamyalgia was thought to be a rare side effect of taking tryptophan regularly, but now the Food and Drug Administration (FDA) believes the disease was caused by contaminates in the manufacturing process. Just to be safe, however, the FDA outlawed health food stores from selling tryptophan tablets to the general public. Only physicians can prescribe the chemical supplement now.

Should you ask your doctor for tryptophan? Taking any chemical supplement is a gamble. However, it probably won't hurt you and you may notice a small improvement in your sleep if you take the pills as recommended. On the other hand, any improvement may be what scientists call a "placebo effect." If you believe the pills will work, then you may convince yourself your sleep is getting better. The best advice is to avoid any chemical supplements to help you sleep. While the research findings on the effectiveness of tryptophan is mixed, the research on the effectiveness of the :60 Second behavior change strategies in chapters 7 and 8 definitely is not. In other words, your chances of improving your sleep are much better if you develop good sleep habits. Eating a balanced diet that includes the recommended daily amounts of milk, eggs and fish will ensure that your body and brain are getting the right amount of tryptophan.

Problems with Long-term Use of Sleeping Pills

Like most medications, sleeping pills were designed to be used on a short-term basis only. Despite this, many people take sleeping pills for months or even years. They may not use them every night, but they rely on them as their only way of coping with insomnia. Recent research indicates that sleeping pills are not as effective in the long-term management of chronic sleep problems as the non-drug :60 Second techniques in this book. Studies have found that individuals prescribed sleeping pills improve their sleep faster, but the initial benefits wear off over time. People who follow a self-management program show slower improvement, but it is better maintained over time. In short, the benefits of self-management last longer, because people are shown how to improve their sleep on their own.

Moreover, taking sleeping pills can put your health at risk for other problems. It can be dangerous to combine sleeping medications with other drugs such as alcohol, muscle relaxants, narcotic analgesics (e.g., Tylenol with codeine) and antidepressants. Most sleeping pills may also cause you to feel tired and less alert during the daytime. Your ability to function in everyday activities may become impaired, putting you at risk for accidents. Recent studies indicate that sleeping pills can also cause memory problems.

Sleep Medications: Drawbacks & Health Risks

- "Hangover" effects the next day
- Increased Stage 2 (light) sleep at the expense of decreased deep (restorative) sleep
- Impairs daytime functioning (sedation, reduced alertness and attention span, reaction time decreased), increasing your risk for accidents and injuries
- Increased risks if combined with other depressants such as alcohol
- Tolerance builds with prolonged use (after as little as two weeks)
- Mild to moderate memory impairment

With sleep medications, there is also the risk that you could develop a tolerance to a sleeping pill so that you have to keep increasing the dose to get the same effect. This happens because most sleeping pills lose their potency with repeated usage. The degree of tolerance that develops depends on a number of factors: the specific medication, pattern of usage and the individual. The following table shows you ways to improve your sleep without using sleeping pills.

:60 Second Ways of Improving Your Sleep		
Goal	**Can a Sleeping Pill Do This?**	**Other, Drug Free Ways**
Get to sleep faster	Yes.	Try sleep restriction (chapter 6) Try relaxation exercises (chapter 9)
Reduce awakenings	Yes, if you take a long-acting one.	Avoid napping; use sleep restriction Reduce caffeine; quit smoking
Deepen your sleep	No, most pills reduce the amount of deep sleep you get.	Exercise every day Avoid napping
Have a more consistent sleep routine	No, most people take pills as needed, in response to poor sleep. Many people over-sleep on these medications.	Follow the stimulus control rules; Get up at same time every morning
Better quality of sleep	Not always.	All of the :60 Second techniques in this book

How to Reduce or Eliminate Use of Sleep Medications

There are important considerations to keep in mind as you try to successfully reduce or eliminate your sleep medications:

1. **Gradually reduce** your use of any sleep medication. You should never stop taking sleep medication suddenly (go "cold turkey"), because this can result in "rebound insomnia" and other withdrawal symptoms. Rebound insomnia is when you experience sleep problems even worse than before you started taking the medication. It happens because your body gets so used to taking the sleeping pills that when they are removed suddenly, your body doesn't know how to sleep without them.

In addition to rebound insomnia, sudden discontinuation of sleeping pills can make you feel anxious. Some people also experience dizziness, nausea, vomiting, tremors and cold spells. The severity of withdrawal symptoms depends on the individual person and on the type of medication, the dosage and pattern of usage.

2.   Establish a **personalized** withdrawal schedule with weekly goals. This is best done in collaboration with your physician. You should be careful about changing medications on your own, without a professional's knowledge or advice. The schedule should take into consideration the specific medication, dosage currently being taken and your ultimate goal (which may be reduction as opposed to elimination of the drug).

It may take up to two months to completely wean off a medication such as a benzodiazepine. A proper withdrawal schedule should have you reduce your original dose each week by about 25 percent. In the latter part of the withdrawal, you will start taking the medication on fewer nights each week and therefore have nights when you don't take any medication. It is vitally important that you take the medication as scheduled and not as you need it. In other words, you may take a pill on some nights you don't feel you need it and take nothing on a potentially "bad" night.

3.   Use the :60 Second strategies in this manual on a regular basis *before* you cut back on your sleep medication. When you first begin reducing your sleep medications, your sleep may seem to get worse and you may be tempted to increase your medication again to compensate. However, instead of doing this, use a relaxation exercise (as described in the next chapter) to help you get to sleep. The important thing is that you have other strategies at your disposal. One of the main reasons that many people continue to take sleep medications is that they don't know any other methods or techniques to help them with their sleep problems. By the time you have finished studying this manual, you will have an arsenal of good sleep strategies at your command.

PART 3

:60 SECOND RELAXATION AND STRESS MANAGEMENT TECHNIQUES FOR IMPROVED SLEEP

chapter 9

COUNTING SHEEP: IMAGERY-BASED RELAXATION

In this chapter you will:
- *Learn the imagery technique for reducing stressful thoughts at bedtime*
- *Learn how to apply the technique specifically to help you get to sleep*

How Imagery Works

There are many forms of relaxation exercises: progressive muscle relaxation (PMR), autogenics, self-hypnosis and meditation, to name a few. Imagery relaxation, also known as visualization, is a special form of relaxation therapy that has proven especially helpful for people who have difficulty sleeping. It differs from overall body relaxation methods in that it uses cognitive (thought-focused) relaxation cues. Imagery works by helping your mind get to sleep along with your body. Your mind controls your thoughts and feelings, as well as necessary bodily functions such as sleeping. Most available research now suggests that a state of mental relaxation rather than physical relaxation is more important for getting to sleep. To sleep, you must turn your mind off or at least put it into a state of relaxation, where your thoughts are free of anxiety-causing images. Many insomniacs complain it is their racing thoughts that keep them awake. They may be physically exhausted when they go to bed, but can't get to sleep because their mind is still wide-awake.

One of the reasons imagery is so effective is that it makes use of the power of the mind's visualization potential. Almost 60 percent of the brain is devoted to processing visual material. Using imagery also has a number of positive effects on your body. The technique can lower your heart rate, blood pressure and reduce tension in your muscles. Emotionally, imagery is also worthwhile, because pleasant images bring on pleasant feelings. If you are upset, anxious or frustrated getting into bed, utilizing pleasurable imagery can evoke more positive emotions. In essence, imagery is a way of diverting attention from negative thoughts about sleeping to a pleasant mental image. Because of this, it is a very effective remedy for sleep performance anxiety. Sustaining a positive image long enough will cause sleep to eventually come.

Imagery is not simply daydreaming or fantasizing. It is an active relaxation procedure that involves your mind more than your muscles. Unlike daydreaming, which is a passive activity, imagery requires active participation in generating and manipulating images. It is a skill that should be practiced every night if possible.

Imagery also can be used to cope with mid-sleep awakenings. Please note that if you are comfortable with another relaxation method such as meditation, you should by no means stop utilizing it, especially if you have been successful in the past in using it to help you get to sleep. However, consider trying the imagery technique and then decide for yourself which is the most effective for inducing sleep faster.

Preparation: Clearing a Space to Relax

Before doing any relaxation exercise, find a relaxing place both for your mind and body in which to perform this new skill. Think of this as your preparation time, similar to what athletes do before a game or competition begins or what musicians do to get ready for a performance. Clearing a physical space can be as simple as creating a bedroom environment that is quiet and free from distraction. If necessary, clear up any clutter in your bedroom if you think an untidy room would bother you. Turn off the television, radio and any other noise-making appliances. You should not use imagery with music in the background, even if you find the music soothing. The music will distract you from your goal of trying to focus on the images in your mind.

If you have a bed partner, you might want to explain to him or her what your needs are when trying to practice the skill of imagery. You should stress the importance of having a quiet bedroom environment. If your partner insists on watching television or reading in bed, you may have to be assertive and ask him or her to hold off from these activities or go to another room.

Now, clear a mental space for yourself. You may be used to mentally hashing and rehashing your problems when trying to get to sleep at night. By doing this you sink deeper into your problems without solving them and make yourself more anxious (and sleep deprived) in the process. The act of worrying can be like a snowball rolling down a hill—the farther down it goes, the more snow it picks up and the bigger it gets. Anxiety can be like that too—the more you worry about your problems, the more anxious you get, not only about the problems themselves, but about the process of worrying as well. Being anxious in itself is anxiety-provoking!

Reduce your anxiety by trying to distance yourself from your problems, at least temporarily. Don't confuse this with running away from difficulties or ignoring them. That wouldn't be helpful either. Rather, take a break and stand back from your anxieties for the period of time you are practicing imagery. Try to imagine yourself standing five yards from your problems, which you could picture as stacks of papers on the ground. Or, imagine yourself setting down that heavy burden you are carrying on your shoulders (picture a large uncomfortable sack that you put on the ground next to you). Give yourself permission to feel good and take a rest. Remember, you're not avoiding your problems or responsibilities, but merely taking a mini-vacation from them.

Practice Imagery Exercises

Next, try two brief but vivid imagery scenes. Get into a comfortable position and read each scene slowly. Then close your eyes and try to imagine the scene as vividly as possible. If you want, you can read the scene slowly out loud and tape record yourself. You can then play it back. Review each scene until you feel as though you are actually in it. When you have achieved this, move onto the step-by-step instructions for the full imagery technique.

Brief Imagery Scene #1

Imagine yourself standing in the middle of a room painted completely in a pleasant shade of green. The walls are green, the floor is green and the ceiling is green. The green reminds you of a tranquil forest. You notice the room is empty except for a single table. On the table is a tall pitcher of iced tea. Suddenly you feel very thirsty. You walk over to the table and grab the pitcher with both hands. You tip the pitcher to your mouth and take a drink of iced tea. You enjoy the sweet lemony taste. The liquid spills over the sides of your mouth and down your shirt.

Brief Imagery Scene #2

Imagine you are standing next to a running stream. It is springtime and the ice has just melted through to the water. The water is deep and swift. It looks cool and refreshing. You can see the rocks at the bottom of the stream. Now imagine that any negative thoughts you have are objects floating down the stream. They float by you and away from you quickly until they are out of your sight completely. If a distracting thought surfaces, let the water take it and whisk it downstream along with any negative thoughts that may enter your mind.

Step-by-step Instructions for Using Imagery

Step 1: Lie in bed and get into a comfortable position. Keep your arms and legs uncrossed. Close your eyes and lie quietly for a few seconds. Clear your mind of stressful thoughts and images.

Step 2: Try to relax all the muscles of your body. If necessary, relax the muscles in your body in groups starting at your toes and working your way up to your head (e.g. toes, feet, legs, thighs, buttocks, abdomen, chest, arms, shoulders, neck, forehead). Avoid tensing your muscles to experience relaxation. Focusing on your lower body first, relax the legs, hips and buttocks. Move up to your upper body and relax your stomach, back, arms and neck. Take a minute to experience the feelings of relaxation and calmness in your body. Focus on the feelings of warmth and heaviness.

Step 3: Do some deep breathing. Take several slow, deep, cleansing breaths. Fill your lungs to capacity with air each time. Wait until you're feeling as relaxed as you can before proceeding. Give yourself praise for getting to this point. Use positive self-statements such as:

"I feel very relaxed."

"I've put away my problems and plans for now."

"I feel calm."

"I won't let any distracting thoughts enter my mind."

"I'm going to sleep well tonight."

"I deserve to feel good."

Step 4: Conjure up a pleasant image that is particularly vivid for you. Make sure that the image has scenes that are calming and are associated with positive emotions. Imagine, for example, a place where you feel safe and comfortable. You can use any image of your own creation. Counting sheep is okay, but I'm sure there are more pleasant images you can choose from. Just make sure that any image you create contains sufficient details to keep you occupied for ten to fifteen minutes.

If you are having trouble creating a positive image, there are two sample images described on the next two pages. Read the description of each image several times and commit it to memory before getting into bed. Note that each series of dots (…) indicates a pause of ten to twenty seconds that you should inject into a scene. This is to give you a moment to enjoy the image. Don't rush!

Step 5: Don't force yourself to concentrate on the scene. Let the images come as naturally as possible. Try not to get frustrated if the image is not as vivid as you initially hoped. Imagery is a skill that must be practiced. In time, your images will become more vivid, more detailed and will conjure up more positive experiences.

Step 6: Be creative in your use of adjectives when conjuring up details of the image. Images with vivid colors, sounds and physical sensations are the most powerful. If you use the same image a number of times, try to experience new details of the image.

Step 7: Keep the image in your mind for at least fifteen minutes. Estimate the passage of time in your head; don't clock-watch. You should not open your eyes at all. At times, intrusive thoughts may come into your mind. You should try not to focus on them or let them go beyond the awareness level. Rather, let them pass and continue to focus on your image.

Full Imagery Scene #1

It is summer. You are walking on a beach alone…You are the only person for miles. It is almost dusk and the sun is setting. The sky, which was a deep blue only an hour ago, is now slowly turning yellow and orange…There are still clouds in the sky. They are billowy and soft like pillows. You remember how hot it was earlier in the day. The temperature is still warm…You feel calm and pleasant inside. The sand feels cool beneath your bare feet. Each foot sinks a little into the soft sand as you walk along the beach. You take a minute to stand still and feel the cool sand between your toes. You wiggle your toes to savor the softness of the sand.

Turning toward the ocean, you can smell the salt water. The fresh salt breeze blows gently against your face…warms your nose…It feels cool and refreshing…You look out toward the sea and spy a lone sailboat on the horizon. Its red sail is fully raised. The sailboat is slowly moving east. You see the wake it leaves in the water as it moves along.

Looking at the sky, the setting sun looks like a bright orange ball. It colors the sky with shades of orange, yellow and pink…Your eyes follow the sky down until it meets the horizon. You notice the rippling reflection of the warm colors in the water. It looks like the water is a giant mirror reflection of everything above.

You walk to the edge of the water and let the tide rush over your toes. The water feels cool and refreshing. As you walk, your feet sink into the wet sand. All is quiet, calm and peaceful. The only sounds you hear are the waves of the ocean as they roll against the shore. You notice the rhythm of the waves as they wash up on the beach. The sound is soothing and relaxing…Your whole body is calm and relaxed.

You feel warm inside. You sit down on the beach in the sand…The warmth cradles your body as you settle in…Closing your eyes, you tune out all your thoughts and focus on the sounds and smells of the ocean surf. You feel warmer and heavier…The place you have made for yourself in the sand is cozy and comfy. You lie back and rest your head in a pillow of soft white sand…The gentle breeze blows around your head…You can think of no other place in the world you would rather be right now—no other way you would rather feel…You are absolutely calm and comfortable…The gentle rhythm of the surf carries you deeper into relaxation…Your whole body is relaxed and your mind is calm and clear…Sleep is coming on—you can feel it overtake your body…Slowly you begin to drift off.

Full Imagery Scene #2

You are at the top of a staircase…Notice what the staircase looks like…Does it have a railing?…Is there carpet on the stairs?…Imagine that you start to descend the staircase one step at a time as you count down from 10…with each step, you find yourself becoming more relaxed and more tired.
…10…getting ready to be completely relaxed;
…9…8…becoming more relaxed; your steps become slower as you descend;
…7…6…feeling more and more relaxed, very comfortable, extremely calm;
…5…4…feeling so calm and relaxed; you can see the bottom of the staircase now;
…3…2…1…you have reached the bottom; you take a deep cleansing breath…

Imagine there is a path that starts at the bottom of the staircase…You start to walk slowly down this path…The path is winding and narrow…You can't see much on either side of the path, but you feel very safe and content…This is a familiar place you have been before…You can't remember quite where this path takes you, but feel the gentle anticipation of arriving soon…You notice how clean the air smells…You look up and see the sky is a deep shade of blue.

You walk along the path until you encounter a special place of yours…Perhaps it is a favorite vacation destination…a tranquil forest…a safe place you remember from childhood…It is a place that gives you fond memories and warm feelings…Picture yourself in the special place…What do you see?…Are you alone?...Are you inside or outside?...Notice the colors and sounds of the place...What do you hear? Is it quiet?

Take a few minutes to enjoy your special place...You are in no rush to leave...You can stay as long as you want...You feel completely relaxed here...Calm...Serene... Stress-free...You continue to breath evenly, deeply and slowly as you prepare to leave.

You are ready to leave...Remind yourself that you can come back any time that you want to...You head back along the path that brought you here...Retrace your footsteps...You feel like you are returning from a vacation...You have just taken a mini-vacation from your problems...

You reach the bottom of the staircase...You start to climb up the staircase slowly and calmly. With each step you feel more and more relaxed...
1...very relaxed...2...still relaxed;
3...4...take a few deep cleansing breaths;
5...6...7...almost at the top of the staircase;
8...9...10...now you are back in your bedroom, feeling very relaxed and ready for sleep...

Common Problems During Imagery Relaxation
Lack of confidence in producing mental images. You don't need great imagination or superior creativity to practice producing mental images. Anyone can do imagery. All that is required is motivation and a little patience. You may be used to having a lot of negative or stress-provoking images occupy your thoughts, especially when trying to get to sleep at night. If this is the case, you should begin by practicing simple, short, positive images before proceeding to longer detailed ones. Use your first attempts to build up your confidence in producing mental images.
Frustration and increased anxiety. You may have difficulty learning to concentrate on imagery at first. Frustration will only serve to increase your tension and arousal level. If you feel yourself getting frustrated, stop working on the present image and switch to a simpler one.
Concentration fading. You may get distracted by other thoughts and feelings. If you are still having difficulty, try focusing on your breathing

for a while. Breathe slowly and deeply. Count each inhale and exhale: "Inhale one... exhale two... inhale three... exhale four."

Focusing on the outcome and not enjoying the experience. Don't fall into the trap of focusing on falling asleep so much that you keep yourself awake in the process. Imagery should be pleasurable no matter what the end result. The more you think about trying to fall asleep, the more aroused you will get. Try to put those thoughts aside and give yourself permission to relax with some pleasant images.

:60 Second Tips for Using Imagery

1. If you are using other relaxation techniques—meditation, for example—for daytime stress, it may be helpful to reserve your use of imagery to cope with sleep problems. One reason to keep your daytime and nighttime relaxation techniques separate is that it will be beneficial to build a strong association between your use of imagery and getting to sleep. That is, you want to reach the point in your program where the mere process of using the technique will make you sleepy.

2. It is important to use imagery every night until you have mastered the technique. You should use it even if you feel you don't need it. In fact, these nights are the most important nights to use imagery. You want to build up the association between imagery and falling asleep. Another reason is that during training, your goal is to build confidence in using imagery to get to sleep. Having a series of nights when it is easy to get to sleep is a great way to build confidence.

3. You can intensify sensory impressions using these techniques: *The more details, the better.* Start with the general and move to the specific. For example, if you imagine an apple, picture more than a simple, round apple. Think of the irregular shape most apples have. Imagine the contours on the skin of the apple and the change in color across its surface.
Be creative in the use of colors. Change the colors of your images. Move beyond using the primary colors (red, green, blue) and experiment with more interesting colors (e.g., fuchsia, lime-green, turquoise).
Add movement. Who says your images have to be motionless? Make

them move or make yourself move if you are imagining a scene with you in it.

Add depth. Create a foreground, middle ground and background to add depth.

Use all five senses. You don't have to stick with only visual images. You can also imagine sounds, smells and the feel of your images. For example, imagine the crisp sound of biting into your apple, the sweet and tart taste of it, the juice running down your chin, etc.

4. Always give yourself praise and use positive self-statements such as:

"I feel quiet."   "I've succeeded with this before."
"I am able to feel relaxed."   "I am doing well."
"I will be asleep soon."   "I can do this, I'm doing this now."

5. Above all, enjoy the experience! Imagery should be a pleasant experience. Using it to help you fall asleep is only one application of imagery. Don't focus on the end result. You should enjoy imagining a scene and enjoy the relaxing respite imagery provides.

chapter 10

MIND OVER MATTER: YOUR THOUGHTS AND SLEEP

In this chapter you will:
- *Explore how your thoughts and feelings affect your sleep*
- *Examine your attitudes and beliefs about sleep*
- *Challenge sleep-interfering beliefs by examining the evidence behind them and developing more realistic beliefs.*

Exploring Your Sleep Mind-set

Let's explore how your thoughts, attitudes and beliefs affect the quality of your sleep. Although we will focus on negative or stress-related thoughts about sleep, the techniques described in this chapter can be used with virtually any disturbing or anxiety causing thoughts that keep you awake at night. The ideas and research of Dr. Charles Morin of Laval University have been instrumental in this area. Dr. Morin was one of the first researchers to recognize how big a role our thoughts and feelings have in determining the quality of our sleep. The process of sleep is, after all, controlled by our brain and not by our body. It makes sense that how we choose to think about sleep will have a big impact on how well we sleep.

Lying in bed at night awaiting sleep is a time when many negative thoughts can come to us. Since there are no activities to distract us, it is the one time of day when we are completely alone with our thoughts. It is also a time when we use our thoughts to talk to ourselves ("self-talk") and address the issues we have been too busy to think about during the day. Many bad sleepers come to associate their bed with places to worry. One patient referred to his bed as the "battleground".

> For most of his adult life, Patrick took his worries to bed with him. He would lie in bed ruminating about the day's activities, usually focusing on negatives (a disagreement with his boss that day, for example.) With his eyes closed, Patrick would replay scenes from the day and worry about mistakes he thought he had made. He could easily imagine how things would be worse the next day or in the future. His worrying was extremely unproductive. It would take him over an hour to fall asleep and then he would wake up several times during the night with the same worries. In the morning he would wake up feeling tired and miserable and dreading going to work.

Living with chronic sleep problems can also lead people to develop many beliefs and assumptions, often erroneous, about why they are sleeping so poorly. This is understandable if you continually have stressful thoughts about the situation. It also is not uncommon for poor sleepers to feel a sense of profound helplessness over their insomnia.

Stressful thoughts about sleep can lead to negative emotions like feelings of tension or anxiety, which can increase your arousal level. It is a well-known fact that when under stress the body reacts in predictable ways. A typical stress response looks like this:

- muscle tension increases
- heart rate increases
- blood pressure rises

We call this the "fight or flight" response. It is caused by a surge of adrenalin into the blood stream causing physical and mental arousal. As we discussed in chapter 2, some people are more sensitive to the arousal caused by stress. Because stressful thoughts lead to physical arousal, it is easy for a vicious cycle of negative emotions and continued poor sleep quality to develop. People sometimes engage in this pattern of stressful thinking without being aware of it. For example, out of habit they may consistently focus on the negative aspects of a situation or belittle their accomplishments. Focusing on the negative all the time is a little like wearing blinders—you neglect to see the positive aspects of situations or fail to recognize solutions when they present themselves. The challenge is to find ways of breaking this pattern and to engage in more realistic, positive self-talk.

The first step in breaking the pattern is to spend some time monitoring your negative "self-talk" about sleep itself. Your attitudes toward sleep can influence how you act on your sleep disturbances and they can create uncomfortable emotional states such as anxiety and depression. Keeping an open mind and adopting healthier mental and emotional attitudes toward sleep can help you become a better sleeper.

:60 Second Technique for Changing Sleep-interfering Thoughts

Next we will put into effect a step-by-step process for recognizing and then changing negative or self-defeating sleep thoughts. You will learn, for example, how to change unhealthy sleep thoughts into more positive attitudes toward sleep. Although these techniques only take a short time to learn, the actual process of changing negative, automatic self-talk will likely take much longer. The instructions are designed as a quick introduction to the process of monitoring and re-thinking some of your self-talk about sleep. Your short-term goal is to become more aware of negative self-talk and the importance of challenging some long-held assumptions about sleep and the effects of sleep loss. Here is a brief overview of the steps, followed by more in-depth explanations.

Step 1: Identify your attitudes and beliefs that are interfering with your sleep. Identify your use of any thinking "biases" that are driving your beliefs.

Step 2: Examine the consequences of holding on to such beliefs.

Step 3: Challenge the truthfulness of each belief system. Determine if the belief is one based on fact or one based on a biased way of thinking.

Step 4: Replace negative self-talk with more accurate thinking ("thinking straight"). This may be as simple as giving yourself permission to consider different interpretations of your problem, without necessarily coming up with the "correct" one.

Steps 1 & 2—Becoming Aware of Your Negative Self-Talk About Sleep

According to Dr. Morin, negative self-talk about sleep itself can be grouped into five general categories. Your own attitudes may not fit into all five categories, so go through them and find the ones that apply to you. Don't get too caught up in labeling your attitudes. Rather, use the opportunity to examine what your belief system is in relation to your attitudes and how these attitudes affect your sleep.

At the core of each self-statement is an underlying belief or assumption that defines the thinking behind the attitude. Underlying some of your attitudes and beliefs may be various "cognitive distortions." A cognitive distortion is simply a tendency to view events in a biased or unrealistic way. In a sense, they "distort" the way in which you look at things, sometimes keeping you from seeing alternative ways of viewing your sleep problem. A list of common cognitive distortions is also shown.

With a little effort, you will be able to recognize the signs that your self-talk may be negative or self-defeating. At first, you may feel that your self-talk is not negative or that it has nothing to do with your sleep problem. Many of the things we say to ourselves seem automatic and unavoidable when in certain situations. Thoughts may pop into our minds so quickly that we don't have time to consider them. You don't want to have to second-guess every thought that comes into your mind. Here are five signs that your self-talk is negative and self-defeating:

1. You start believing that thoughts are facts. For example, you imagine the worst and believe it will happen just because you are thinking it.
2. Your thoughts bring unpleasant emotional reactions such as feelings of depression, anxiety, distress, anger, guilt and irritability. Do an "emotion check."

3. You have physical symptoms of stress such as increased heart rate, temperature changes (cold clammy hands is a sign of stress) and increased muscle tension in your forehead, back and neck. Ask yourself, "What was I thinking that caused that physical response?"
4. Your predictions about future events rarely come true. For example, when you expect to have a bad day because you didn't sleep well, but your day turns out fine.
5. You are much harder on yourself than you would be on others. You may be your own worst enemy and expect more from yourself than you expect from others.

Distorted Ways of Thinking about Sleep
1. **All-or-nothing thinking.** You see things in black and white categories. For example, if your performance falls short of perfect, you see yourself as a total failure. Example: *I must have eight hours of sleep every night. Anything less is not acceptable.*

2. **Overgeneralization.** You use a single negative event as proof of always being defeated. Example: *I tried relaxation last night to get to sleep, but it didn't work; nothing will help me.*

3. **Filtering events.** You wear blinders and only see the negative aspects of a situation. The glass is always half empty to you. Example: *I woke up twice last night and had difficulty getting back to sleep each time. My whole night's sleep was ruined.*

4. **Ignoring the positive and belittling your accomplishments.** You don't acknowledge positive events when they happen. Example: *I had a few nights of pretty good sleep, but I still don't sleep as well as my husband.*

5. **Fortune telling.** You predict the future will turn out badly. If given the choice between a positive outcome and negative one, you predict the negative one will happen. Example: *What's the point in trying? I know my sleep will never get any better.*

6. **Blowing things out of proportion (catastrophizing).** You usually believe the absolute worst possible outcome will happen (you "catastrophize"). Example: *I was sleeping well for over two weeks, but then I had a night of complete sleeplessness. My progress is ruined; all my hard work was for nothing.*

7. **Emotional reasoning.** You assume that if you feel something strongly, then it must be true. Example: *I need those sleeping pills. I could never give them up.*

8. **"Shoulding" all over yourself.** You have high expectations of yourself which you reinforce with "should" and "should not" statements. When you don't achieve what you expect of yourself, you feel guilty or inadequate. Example: *I shouldn't be getting out of bed so often at night. It will wake up my wife and kids.*

Five Categories of Negative Self-talk about Sleep

1. **Being unrealistic about how much sleep you need.** Many insomniacs believe that they need a full eight hours of sleep every night to function normally. They also assume that all people need the same amount of sleep every night.

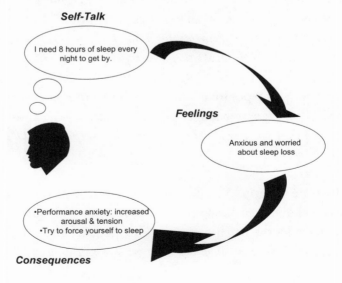

2. **Attributing poor sleep to uncontrollable factors.** Do you blame your insomnia on physical factors or other things out of your control? Unfortunately, by doing this, you are ignoring the role that faulty sleep habits and other psychological factors have in maintaining poor sleep quality.

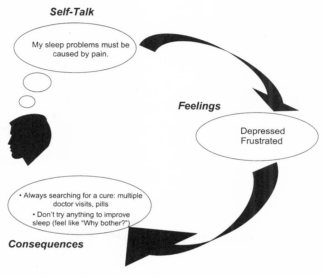

3. **Making mountains out of molehills.** Do you have a tendency to exaggerate how much your sleep problems affect your peace of mind? By doing this, you may be maintaining the vicious cycle of bad feelings and poor sleep.

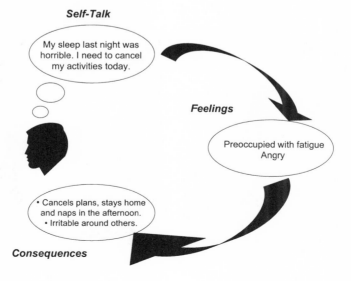

4. **Feeling that sleep controls you.** The underlying belief here is that you see sleep as being externally controlled and yourself as a helpless victim of poor sleep. Unfortunately, holding this belief can sustain your feelings of powerlessness.

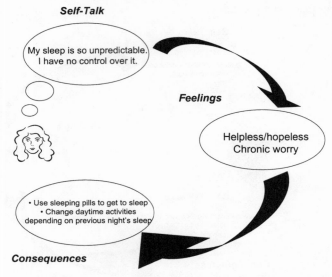

5. **Not wanting to give up old habits, even when they don't work well.** Are you holding on to old beliefs about sleep-promoting activities? Consequently, you may be engaging in ineffective coping strategies such as staying in bed even when you can't get to sleep.

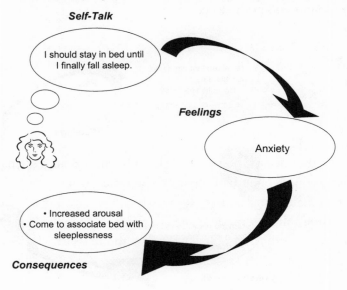

Step 3—Disputing Sleep Interfering Self-talk

The best way to change negative self-talk is to examine the actual evidence (the facts) supporting the underlying belief. By challenging the underlying belief, you open the door for other attitudes to emerge. You also disrupt the perpetual cycle of bad thoughts, negative emotions and poor sleep.

Remember that *thoughts are not facts.* Therefore, to challenge your negative self-talk, you need to check the accuracy of the evidence you have available to you. When possible, try to dispute the evidence in favor of more realistic evidence. Use these dispute statements to help you:

"Do I know for certain that _____will happen?"

"Am I 100 percent sure of these consequences?"

"What evidence do I have that _____will happen?"

"Can I predict the future all the time?"

"What is the worst that could happen?"

"Could there be any other explanations?"

"Is _____really so important?"

In the next few pages we will look closer at the five categories of negative self-talk about sleep and learn ways to challenge the underlying beliefs with actual evidence.

Step 4—Thinking Straight

By challenging some of your negative self-talk you can start to look at alternative interpretations of your situation. Remember, it is not important that you always find the "correct" solution or "the answer" to your problems. What is important is that you allow yourself to look at things in a different way when you feel stuck. One of the most damaging aspects of negative self-talk is not the thoughts themselves or whether or not they are true, but the emotional response they bring out in you. Feeling bad most of the time can be pretty draining. The unfortunate thing is that after a while, these feelings start to become a routine thing, sometimes to the point that you can't remember ever feeling any other way. This is one of the reasons why changing negative self-talk can be a challenge.

Replacing negative thoughts with positive self-talk is not always easy, but it is possible. Initially, you should strive to find as many alternative ways of looking at your problem as possible. You don't have to do all the work on your own. Ask your spouse or a friend for their opinions. Try to test the validity of your assumptions with personal "experiments." For example, test your assumption that you need to nap everyday in the afternoon by avoiding napping for a while and seeing how you feel.

When you start coming up with new interpretations of your problem, phrase them in the form of positive self-statements and say them back to yourself. Then say them out loud to yourself and to others. Do an emotion check while doing this. Simply ask yourself how you are feeling when you say these things. The following table provides some examples of positive self-statements you can use to dispute erroneous beliefs about sleep.

Please remember that positive self-talk is not to be confused with the "power of positive thinking" or having mindless happy thoughts (for example, saying to yourself, *The world is a wonderful place with no bad people in it*). You don't want to delude yourself and ignore your problems. Rather, the goal is to have accurate, realistic and open-minded self-talk. Be just as critical of your positive self-talk as your negative thoughts.

Thinking Straight About Your Sleep Problems

Sleep-interfering Thought	Actual Evidence & Other Explanations	Positive Self-statements You Can Use Instead
I need eight hours of sleep every night.	People differ in the amount of sleep they need; the range is from four to ten hours in the general population.	"Just because my husband needs eight hours of sleep, doesn't mean I do."
	The amount of deep or quality sleep is more important than the total amount of sleep.	"It's not how much I sleep that is important; it is the quality of my sleep."
	Some famous people (Jay Leno, Thomas Edison, Martha Stewart) are short sleepers.	"I'm one of those people who gets by on less sleep."

Sleep-interfering Thought	Actual Evidence & Other Explanations	Positive Self-statements You Can Use Instead
My sleep problems must be caused by pain.	Lots of people with pain have only mild problems sleeping. And then there are some people with pain who don't have any sleep disturbances.	"Sleep disturbances are not an all-or-nothing event with pain."
	Most people do have good nights of sleeping that are not related to changes in pain level.	"Just because I have pain doesn't mean I have to suffer from poor sleep every night."
	Regardless of the medical reason, there are always psychological factors that affect sleep quality.	"Maybe I can't stop the pain, but I can modify and even eliminate the other things contributing to my sleep problems."
A night of poor sleep is going to ruin my day.	Do you always function poorly after a bad night of sleep?	"What is the worst that can happen? I may feel a little tired, but if I keep busy I probably won't notice it."
	Most people experience only mild impairment in their functioning after being completely deprived of sleep. After sleep loss, people's performance goes down slightly on simple, boring tasks (e.g., adding numbers), but they do fine on more complex or interesting activities.	"I know that if I do something boring, I'll start to feel tired and want to have a nap. Therefore, I'm going to find activities that will kept my mind active and interested."
	The biggest effect of sleep loss is on mood. However, even this is more likely to be related to the original cause of the sleepless night (e.g., stress) rather than sleep loss.	"Sleep loss tends to make me grouchy and irritable, but I can change that. I'll make an effort to watch my mood and try to be more cheerful instead."
	You can achieve most of your restorative sleep in three to four hours.	"It's more important to get three to four hours of continuos sleep rather than eight hours of broken-up sleep."

Sleep-interfering Thought	Actual Evidence & Other Explanations	Positive Self-statements You Can Use Instead
I didn't sleep well last night; I will have to take a nap today to catch up on my lost sleep.	Taking a nap will likely interfere with your sleep at night since it is like starting your sleep period early.	"Do I know for certain that I need a nap? I've made it through other days without a nap."
	If you prolong your nap until you go to bed, you'll go to bed sleepy and sleep more that night.	"If I have a nap, I may rob myself of deep sleep tonight"
		"Is having a sixty minute nap so important to my well-being?"
I can never predict if I will have a good or bad night of sleep.	Feeling like your sleep controls you leads to frustration, more anxiety and a tendency to focus on feelings of sleeplessness rather than sleepiness. This can be more harmful than the actual loss of sleep.	"So I can't always control my sleep all the time—I'm not going to let this get me stressed.
	Your nighttime sleep is affected by daytime activities, thoughts and feelings. Learn to recognize these relationships and focus your attention on those things under your control.	[In the morning] "Today, I will try to not let things upset me so that I will be calm when I go to bed."

:60 Second Techniques for Managing Stress

There are other coping techniques you can use throughout the day to help you deal with stressful thoughts. One thing you should recognize is that it is not always possible to solve a problem right away. Some problems require time to resolve. Other problems can't be solved directly by you; they may require the input of other people. However, just because you can't solve a problem right away, does not mean you can't manage the problem. Every problem can be managed so that the amount of stress it causes you is minimized. The ability to manage problems effectively is a skill that can be learned.

Some General Techniques for Managing Stress

Concentrate on one problem at a time. When thinking about problems, many people increase worry and anxiety by constantly shifting from one problem to the next. This makes it seem like you have twice as many problems or that you are going in circles all the time trying to solve them. You cannot resolve a problem by only thinking about it for a few seconds or minutes at a time.

Focus on the most manageable problem first. Start with either the problem that is giving you the most distress or the one that you think you can resolve the easiest. Concentrate on that problem to the exclusion of all other problems. Sort out as many details and issues as possible concerning the problem.

Plan your worrying time. If you are going to worry, you might as well make it a productive time. Therefore, rather than worry about your problems in bed when you cannot do anything about them, set a specific time and place (e.g., 2:30 P.M., at home in the living room) during the day to do your worrying. Designate a thirty-minute worry period. Focus on only one problem at a time and try to make the time productive by coming up with some options for dealing with the problem. Next time you cannot get to sleep because you are thinking about your problems, remind yourself that you have set some time out the next day to worry.

As a suggestion, make your worrying time the time you normally nap. Don't sleep, however, and don't lie in bed; rather, sit up and do your worrying. This will help you curtail napping.

Try relaxation exercises. Use some of the relaxation tips in the previous chapter to cope with stress during the day.

Imagine the worst outcome and develop a plan to deal with it (de-catastrophizing). Sometimes it is the fear of the unknown that can be troublesome and anxiety-provoking. When faced with a big problem, we don't always like to think about the consequences or the "worst-case scenario." It seems enough to know that something bad will happen without thinking about the details. This is an example of emotional thinking, since we assume that the consequences will be as bad as the feelings we assign to them. By not thinking about the details of the worst scenario, however, you deny yourself the opportunity to develop a plan to deal with it.

Therefore, imagine the worst possible outcome to your problem. In your mind, map out the sequence of events that would occur and the consequences of each. Engulf yourself in as much detail as you can stand. Do this several times until you are completely bored with the problem. Now, develop your plan for dealing with the consequences. Although going through it will not be pleasant, remind yourself that the consequences will likely be short-lived and under your control. Remind yourself that you have probably gotten through worse times before.

After you've done this exercise, one of two things will happen: (1) the worst doesn't happen, in which case you will be relieved, or (2) the worst does happen, in which case you have your plan prepared in advance to minimize the impact. It will still be difficult, but not as difficult as if you had not prepared.

> *Sally spent several sleepless nights worrying about her performance appraisal at work. She had struggled in her job the last couple of months due to being unfamiliar with a new computer system. She had missed an important deadline because of this. Sally was afraid of what her supervisor would say to her on Friday. Even the thought of the performance evaluation made her anxious. The night before the evaluation she had had enough and decided to fight back against her anxiety. She got out of bed and thought about the worst case scenario. She imagined her supervisor would comment on her performance and question whether she had the skills to work with this new computer system. She imagined her supervisor saying things like "I am starting to wonder, Sally, if you are the right person for this position." Sally then thought of several good responses. She knew she could learn the new system if she had the proper training. In the morning she planned to look up when the next course would be starting and would offer to take it on her own time if her supervisor wanted. She felt better after planning this and slept through the night for the first time all week.*

Do your worrying on paper and not in your head. By always keeping worries in your mind, it is difficult to get any distance from them. Write out all of the problems that are significant stressors in your life. When you list them down on paper they may look a little more manageable. Try your best to manage your problems on paper.

Write out the possible solutions and brainstorm alternatives. Work at them for an hour. Then when you are done, gather up the papers and put them away. Do this every time you want to work on your problems.

One advantage of doing your worrying on paper is that you have a written record of your thoughts. When worrying, people tend to ruminate or go over and over problems, sometimes thinking of a possible solution but then dismissing it. At times, people think of the same solution many times, but never really develop it into a plan. By thinking on paper, you can review your records and see what ideas you have considered and what ideas you have not. You may discover you had already thought of a solution and forgotten it.

Michael started a journal of his thoughts and worries. When he couldn't sleep at night, he got out of bed and wrote down his thoughts in his journal. He sometimes came up with partial solutions to his problems, which he wrote down. He found this helpful in reducing his anxiety while lying in bed, because he knew he had done some productive worrying on paper.

Stay up all night worrying. If you try the written strategies and fail, then try this: purposely stay up all night worrying. In other words, don't try to distract yourself from your problems, rather give them your undivided attention for the entire night. It is possible that nighttime is your best time to worry. So get up and worry, worry, worry. Just don't do it in bed. Remember, worrying in bed will just turn your bed into the place where you worry instead of the place where you sleep. Therefore, get out of bed, find yourself a new spot in which to worry and go to it!

chapter 11

PROBLEM-SOLVING FOR INSOMNIA

In this chapter you will:

*   *Learn how to use the "S.O.L.V.E." problem-solving technique to deal with insomnia*

:60 Second Problem-Solving Technique

Another problem-solving technique (S.O.L.V.E.) developed by psychologists Thomas D'Zuriella and Marvin Goldfried has been used to resolve many different types of problems. In this section, we'll apply this five-step program specifically to sleep problems.

D'Zuriella and Goldfried define a problem as *a failure to find an effective response.* In other words, it is not the situation, but what you make of it, that determines whether a problem exists. For example, your car not starting one morning when you have to get to work is not necessarily a problem. A problem emerges when you cannot find an alternative way of getting to work on time. A problem can also occur if you employ a response that ends up making the situation worse. For example, trying to fix the car yourself may make the mechanical problem worse in addition to wasting time and causing you to be even later for work.

The S.O.L.V.E. technique goes like this:

> **S**tate your problem
> **O**utline your response
> **L**ist your alternatives
> **V**iew the consequences
> **E**valuate your results

Step-by-Step Problem-Solving Instructions
It will be helpful to use the problem-solving worksheet shown on the last page of this chapter.

Step 1: State Your Problem. Write out your problem on paper. Make sure you phrase it in a way that conforms with the definition of a problem as a failure to find an effective response.
Example: Doug has a problem with daytime napping.
Doug's *incorrect* statement of problem: "I can't help but nap in the afternoon and this interferes with my sleep at night."
Doug's *correct* statement of the problem: "I haven't found the best way to curb my napping habit."

Step 2: Outline Your Response. Describe your *usual* response to the problem (that is, what you do or don't do). You can use the following outline to define in more detail your response. Be sure to include the persons and events that are usually involved.

Example: Doug's daytime napping

Who is involved? (the other people)	Doug: *"I'm the only one involved."*
What happens? (what is done or not done that bothers you)	*I take a nap when I know I shouldn't.*
When does it happen? (time of day, how often, how long it lasts)	*Mid-afternoon every day of the week for about one and one-half hours.*
Where does it happen? (location)	*I nap in my bed.*
How does it happen? (sequence of events, your mood at the time)	*After lunch, I start to feel tired, because I didn't sleep well the night before. Eventually I lie down and fall asleep.*
Why does it happen? (the reasons you or others give for the problem)	*I need to sleep. I need to catch up on the sleep I lost the previous night. If I don't nap, I'll feel terrible.*

Step 3: List Alternative Solutions to the Problem. Do some "brainstorming" and generate a list of alternative strategies or approaches to your problem. Brainstorming means thinking of anything, no matter how crazy or unbelievable it sounds, that

could be a possible solution to your problem. A few guidelines for brainstorming are:

- **Don't be critical of any idea at first.** Just write each one down. Later, you can sort out ideas that are practical from those that are not.
- **The crazier the better.** Open your mind to new things, even if they defy normal logic. Be creative.
- **The more ideas, the better.** Quantity is better than quality, at least at first. The more ideas with which you start, the greater your chances of finding one or two good ones. Therefore, make a long list—a minimum of *ten ideas* is suggested.
- **Worry about the details later.** The how's and why's of each idea are not important. Don't waste time with details until you have narrowed your list down.

Referring back to our napping example, remember that we defined this problem as Doug's inability to find effective ways of coping with the sleepiness that occurs in the daytime. From the outline of Doug's usual response to this problem we see that his naps usually occur in the mid-afternoon and he naps in bed. His interpretation of why it happens is that he feels sleepy and can't resist lying down.

We now want to generate a list of alternative strategies to taking a nap in the afternoon.

Brainstorming Alternatives to Napping

1. Go biking instead of napping.
2. Get wife or roommate to throw cold water in face to stay awake.
3. Drink a pot of coffee or a case of Coke.
4 Plan on doing housework in mid-afternoon.
5. Get a volunteer job that starts at 2:00 P.M. and goes to 5:00 P.M. every day.
6. Make my nap time my "worrying time" instead. Spend this time period focusing exclusively on my most distressing personal problem. Problem solve for solutions or ways of managing the problem.

7. Arrange to meet a friend every afternoon to go for a walk.
8. Replace my bed with a sofa bed that has a time lock that keeps closed all day.
9. Put a sign on my front door that says "Solicitors welcome, especially in the afternoon."
10. Move next to the airport and leave my windows open all day.
11. Have a friend call every day in the afternoon to talk about sports and politics.

Step 4: View the Consequences. Now, go over the list of alternatives to napping and pick out the ones that seem the most promising or appealing. You'll notice that the list contains some ideas that seem outrageous or impractical. On the other hand, they would be solutions to the problem—having water thrown in your face would keep you from taking a nap! Besides, some outrageous ideas contain elements of practicality. Take the water throwing example. Although using water is outrageous, the idea of involving a spouse or friend to help you is not. This one outrageous alternative helped generate a few more alternatives that solicit the support of others in coping with this problem.

Cross out all the ideas that are too unrealistic. Look at the remaining ideas. If you wish, you can combine one or more strategies based on common elements. For example, what #4, 5, 6, and 7 all share is the idea that Doug should plan a regular activity every day in the afternoon when he normally takes a nap. Since it might be impractical or tedious to do the same activity every afternoon, he should construct a weekly schedule with a variety of different activities planned for afternoons.

After combining ideas, you should be down to two or three possibilities. Now you have to think about the consequences of putting each idea into action. In other words, consider the pros and cons of each idea. Things to consider are: how it would make you feel (relieved? more anxious?) and how easy or difficult would it be to make the change long-term?

Write out the pros and cons for each strategy. Decide how much importance you would assign each pro and con. When deciding which strategy to use, you should take into consideration not only the total number of pros and cons for each, but how important they are. Ultimately, you should choose the strategy in which the pros outweigh the cons either in number or in importance.

Step 5: <u>E</u>valuate the Results. Now it is time to act on your choice(s). Put your plan into effect and observe the consequences. What happened? Any surprises? Are you satisfied with the outcome? If not, you go to the next option on your list of alternative strategies. One great thing about this method is that you don't have to limit yourself to just one strategy. Using the S.O.L.V.E. process, you will be able to systematically and logically generate a list of strategies to manage your problem.

Some people criticize this method, arguing that they just end up dealing with their problem in the "same old way" or that they use the most obvious strategy they came up with. Is it a waste of time then? The thing to ask yourself is how confident do you feel about the decision you made? How confident do you think you would have felt with that decision if you had not gone through the problem-solving method and assessed the pros and cons of every alternative?

Making a decision about which you don't feel confident can sometimes create more anxiety than the original problem, especially if you feel that you are making a hasty decision and missing some other possible strategy. By using the S.O.L.V.E. method, you should feel more confident with your decision, because you know that you have used a proven technique to arrive at *the best possible choice given your alternatives.*

Another advantage to this method is that you can do your problem solving on paper rather than in your head. By always thinking about your problem, it is difficult to get any distance from it and look at it objectively. Problems tend to look a little more manageable when they are written out on paper. Remember, do your thinking on paper and not in your head. This way you have a written record of your thinking. When worrying, people tend to ruminate, going over and over problems, sometimes thinking of a possible solution but then dismissing it. By doing problem solving on paper, you can review your records and see what ideas you have considered and what ideas you have not.

Sleep Problem-Solving Worksheet

State your sleep problem:

Outline your typical response

Where do I do it?

When do I do it?

How do I do it?

How do I feel?

What do I want?

List your alternatives (Brainstorming)

1. _____

2. _____

3. _____

4. _____

5. _____

6. _____

7. _____

8. _____

9. _____

10. _____

View the consequences (assess the pros and cons of each alternative)

Pros	Cons	Potential effectiveness (1=least; 5=most)
1. _____	1. _____	_____
2. _____	2. _____	_____
3. _____	3. _____	_____
4. _____	4. _____	_____
5. _____	5. _____	_____
6. _____	6. _____	_____
7. _____	7. _____	_____
8. _____	8. _____	_____
9. _____	9. _____	_____
10. _____	10. _____	_____

Evaluate the result once you have implemented one strategy

What happened?

Were you surprised or was the outcome just what you expected?

Are you happy with the results?

If you are not satisfied with the outcome, try an alternative strategy and re-evaluate when you are finished.

PART 4

SLEEP CONCERNS OF WOMEN, CHILDREN AND ADOLESCENTS

chapter 12

WOMEN AND INSOMNIA

In this chapter you will:
- *Learn about the unique sleep concerns of women*
- *Discover how the menstrual cycle and menopause can affect sleep*
- *Learn tips for improving sleep while coping with the physical changes that occur during and after menopause*

Are women more at risk to develop sleep problems? The answer seems to be yes. Certainly, the data collected from large research studies in the United States and Europe clearly show that women are one and one-half to two times more likely to experience insomnia. Women may be more at risk, particularly when entering menopause. In fact, between 30 percent and 50 percent of women aged forty to sixty years who were going through menopause report having sleep disturbances.[1] However, only about a third of patients raised the issue of poor sleep with their physicians. This suggests that many women do not get treatment for insomnia.

There are many possible explanations for the higher rate of insomnia among women compared to men. One possibility is that men underreport or deny sleep disturbances, but this alone is unlikely to explain the entire difference in the rates of insomnia reported between the sexes. The physiological differences between men and women may be a strong contributing factor, particularly during later life. In addition, there are important lifestyle differences that can contribute to women having more sleep problems than men. In the next few sections, you will learn more about these and some of the other unique sleep concerns of women.

Lifestyle and Social Role Factors

It is important to consider some of the lifestyle factors that may contribute to sleep disturbances in women. The link between stress and sleep problems is clearly established. Do women have more stress? Statistics indicate that women work more hours per week than men. Although women are working outside the home in greater numbers these days, many still find that they do the majority of housework. In addition, they typically assume the major role in child care and child rearing. A woman who works a full day outside the home may find her evening is spent cooking, cleaning and attending to the needs of the children. This is particularly true of single mothers, but also of married women. Consequently, many women find they have much less leisure time than their husbands or their male friends. Many find themselves physically exhausted by the end of the day. Although physical activity is good for sleep, activity to the point of exhaustion can cause disruption to nighttime sleep. Furthermore, many women seem to carry the emotional burdens of their families, which can cause more stress. For example, mothers are often the ones who keep track of family birthdays, anniversaries and do the planning for these and other special occasions. They are also more likely to be the ones to care for sick parents and other relatives.

Another major disruption to a woman's sleep can be the arrival of a baby. New mothers often joke about their lack of nighttime sleep. Fortunately, we live in a more enlightened society now and dads are more inclined to help out with the nighttime care of an infant. Nevertheless, the responsibility of breast-feeding a baby still falls to mom (at least until scientists invent a way for fathers to provide this service). With few exceptions, the first three months of motherhood typically means a chaotic sleeping schedule for the new mother. Even after their babies start to sleep through the night, many women find their sleep remains light and fragmented for quite some time. The experience of having a child seems to make women more sensitive to night noises, especially the cries or stirrings of their young children. Consequently, women seem to have more awakenings than men and are more likely to wake up feeling like they did not get much of the precious deep sleep we all need.

Menstrual Cycle

To understand how the menstrual cycle affects sleep, it may help to briefly review what happens during a normal cycle. In the days leading up to ovulation (known as the follicular phase of the cycle), the levels of the female hormones estrogen and progesterone in the body start to increase. The higher levels of these hormones have an important purpose—to signal the uterus lining to thicken and grow in anticipation of a fertilized egg (this is known as the luteal phase). The midcycle peak of another chemical in the body called luteinizing hormone (LH) triggers the actual release of an egg by the ovaries (ovulation phase). After ovulation, there is another increase in the levels of estrogen and progesterone in the blood in preparation for possible impregnation. If the egg is not fertilized, the levels of sex hormones in the body gradually decline. This is followed by the beginning of menstruation in which the body discharges the endometrial tissue through the vagina.

The process of menstruation causes weekly, even daily, variations in the levels of sex hormones, body temperature and metabolic rate in women. Men, in contrast, maintain the same levels of their sex hormones throughout the month and they experience relatively minor variations in temperature and metabolism. The differences between male and female physiology have made it difficult for researchers to study normal sleep processes. In fact, many of the early studies on human sleep actually excluded women, because researchers felt it was difficult to account for the variations in sleep patterns that were assumed to occur in women throughout their cycles. Complicating the situation is the fact that all women are different. Although the average menstrual cycle is twenty-eight days, the actual length varies quite a bit from woman to woman, as do the specific levels and timing of hormone release during the cycle. Imagine trying to study the sleep of twenty women, all with different cycles, sleep histories and metabolic rates. Studying men seems a whole lot simpler!

Despite the challenges, researchers have managed to piece together what happens to sleep throughout the stages of the menstrual cycle. Sleep is greatly affected by a woman's monthly cycle.[2] Disturbances of sleep during menstruation affect some but not all women. Many women are not aware of any changes in their sleep patterns coinciding with a particular phase of their menstrual cycle. In general, however, many women seem to get the best sleep during the early part of the menstrual cycle when estrogen levels are just starting to rise. Sleep disturbances, if any, are most likely to occur during the latter, premenstrual phase of the cycle. For example, there is an increase in the number of awakenings during the late luteal phase (the last few days before menstruation begins), which coincides with decreased levels of estrogen and progesterone in the body. Some studies show that during this phase, on average, women report taking longer to fall asleep and having poorer sleep quality compared to other times of the month. Other studies have found a decrease in deep (slow-wave) sleep during the premenstruation phase. These effects can occur in healthy women who do not complain of chronic sleep problems. For women who have chronic insomnia, a somewhat different picture emerges. Studies have shown that changes in sleep during the normal menstrual cycle do not add much additional disruption to the sleep of insomniacs. In other words, women with chronic insomnia seem to have poor sleep regardless of their progression through the menstrual cycle.

Sleep changes during the menstrual cycle are highly individual, just as the cycle itself varies from woman to woman. Many women do not notice any changes in their sleep before their periods begin. For other women, the premenstruation phases of their cycles are associated with considerable physical and psychological stress. Premenstrual syndrome (PMS) describes the constellation of symptoms that precede the beginning of menstruation. As a medical condition, PMS is still not well understood. Some researchers attribute PMS to uncomfortable cramps, water retention and heavy vaginal bleeding. However, the experience of PMS varies greatly from woman to woman. Many women do not experience these symptoms, while others show dramatic changes in their mood and general health before menstruation starts. The emotional changes that are typically associated with PMS—namely depression, irritability and anger—can also contribute to sleep disturbances in addition to the physical changes in the body.

Coping with sleep disturbances that are caused by PMS or menstruation itself is really no different from coping with insomnia caused by other things. One coping technique women who do experience sleep disturbances may find particularly helpful is imagery relaxation (chapter 9). Imagery is a good way to distract your thoughts from the anticipatory stress of PMS or the physical discomfort of menstruation. Women who experience highly irregular and uncomfortable periods sometimes get relief by taking birth control pills. The pill seems to help regulate the menstrual cycle and make the physical symptoms of PMS, including insomnia, more tolerable. Despite these benefits, the pill does have risks. It does not protect a woman from sexually transmitted diseases and women who take the pill for long periods have a higher risk for developing breast cancer. If you are considering this option, please talk to your doctor about the advantages and disadvantages of the pill.

Menopause
What is Menopause?
Most women will start menopause sometime between the ages of forty-five and sixty, with fifty-one being the average. If a woman is a smoker, the chances of starting menopause at an earlier age are much greater. Under certain conditions, a woman can enter menopause before the age of forty. For example, having a total hysterectomy—which is sometimes a medical necessity in the case of ovarian tumors or other serious pelvic disease—can lead to premature menopause. Early menopause can also occur in response to acute or prolonged stress, although this is rare.

Normal menopause is actually a gradual process caused by the slowing down of the body's production of estrogen with age. In the year or two before the onset of menopause, a woman will start to have more irregular menstrual cycles. For example, she may miss a period, have very heavy menstruation another month and very little flow the next month. All this is the result of lower levels of estrogen in the body. Many women notice other changes: their sexual desire may fluctuate, hot flashes may start (although you may not recognize them as hot flashes yet), appetite may diminish and, of course, sleep problems may increase. This part of menopause is known as the perimenopause phase and typically will last from one to three years.

The term menopause officially refers to the one-year period starting with the last menstrual cycle. It is during this year that most women find the changes in their bodies to be the most noticeable. Despite the horror stories, menopause for most women is nothing more than another transition in their lives. Women today have more information about menopause and seem to be better prepared for the changes. Like most transitions in life, however, responses are highly individual. For some women, the end of their menstrual cycle can be experienced as a rather significant loss because it signals the end of their childbearing potential. Some change in sexuality is quite normal, but often it is only temporary until the woman and her sexual partner learn how to adapt. Other women may openly embrace the end of having a period, particularly if their menstrual cycles have been very irregular and uncomfortable.

Sleep Problems During Menopause
The sleep disturbances that occur during menopause have been studied quite extensively. It appears that a large number of women—anywhere from 30 percent to 50 percent, depending on the survey—will experience symptoms of insomnia during menopause. Sleep problems generally get worse as women go through the various stages of menopause: pre-menopause, perimenopause, menopause and post-menopause. Of course, women also get older as they go through these stages and sleep generally gets lighter and more fragmented with age. Nevertheless, research has shown that menopause is associated with sleep problems that cannot be solely attributed to age-related changes. Studies in which women going through menopause are compared with pre-menopausal women the same age find that the menopausal women show significantly more sleep disturbances.

Physical or psychological? Of course, the experience of menopause goes beyond the physical changes. It is also a time when some women experience many emotional changes. Although all women are different, menopause for many women can be associated with periods of depression, anxiety, periodic feelings of loss, a change in body image and even decreased self-esteem. Both physical changes and psychological changes can lead to sleep problems and trying to sort out what is causing what is often a challenge. We know that changes in psychological well-being can have a big impact on sleep, particularly if you are the sort of sleeper who takes your stressful thoughts to bed with you. The onset of menopause may happen to coincide with other transitions in a woman's life. Midlife women often find themselves coping with their children leaving home, having to care for their own aging parents, adjusting to a separation, divorce or even the death of their spouse and reentering the work force.

Hot flashes. Research into the physical impact of menopause on sleep has identified hot flashes as being the primary source of sleep disturbances. A typical hot flash is a sudden increase in skin temperature and heart rate, accompanied by a visible flushing of the skin. Sweating is also common. A hot flash has similar physical symptoms to a panic attack, but without the intense rush of anxiety (although many women find hot flashes unsettling and stressful). The average flash lasts about three minutes and then the body starts to cool down. As a woman has more hot flashes, she can generally start to anticipate them. Hot flashes can occur during sleep and some women say that they are awakened by nocturnal flashes. Sleep that is interrupted by hot flashes can be very fragmented (due to many mid-sleep arousals) and lighter than normal. After a night of intermittent hot flashes, most women wake up in the morning feeling like their sleep was not very refreshing.

Not all menopausal women have full-blown hot flashes during sleep. Some get night sweats instead. Night sweats may or may not wake you up, but can be uncomfortable and inconvenient nonetheless. The person who suffers them may not be aware of night sweats until they wake up and find damp sheets and bedclothes. Night sweats are a sign that your internal temperature is irregular during the night. Body temperature normally decreases during the first part of the sleep cycle, reaching its low point around 4:00 or 5:00 A.M. Then it starts to gradually increase as normal waking time approaches. The ups and downs in body temperature caused by hot flashes or night sweat activity can be very disruptive to the sleep cycle. The part of the brain that regulates temperature is closely related to the part that controls sleep, so when one is disrupted it seems to affect the other.

Hormone Replacement Therapy

Hormone replacement therapy has been available for several decades, but in the last ten years we have seen an explosion of information on HRT and more aggressive promotion of it as a form of treatment for menopause. About one in four women choose to take HRT. Some women are feeling pressured to take HRT without knowing the associated risks and the other choices that are available. Please remember that *hormone replacement therapy is a personal choice* and that not all women need to take HRT. In this section, we will briefly explain hormone replacement therapy, the pros and cons of HRT and how it may help if you have insomnia from menopause. For more information on HRT, there are several good books on menopause, including *:60 Second Menopause Management* by Carol Schulz, that will tell you in greater detail what you need to know. You can also talk to your doctor about HRT.

Hormone replacement therapy consists of taking estrogen, progestin or a combination of these two in the form of pills, skin patches or creams. Premarin is the most commonly prescribed estrogen tablet. In the last five years, Premarin has also been one of the three most commonly prescribed medications in the United States, which demonstrates how popular the drug is becoming. There are lots of reasons to take HRT and lots of reasons to be cautious when considering HRT. Please be aware that research on HRT is ongoing, so we do not know everything about the pros and cons of HRT and may not know for several more years. To date, the main advantages of HRT for women seem to be:

• Reduces frequency and severity of hot flashes
• Decreases vaginal dryness, which may improve sexual functioning
• Decreases risk of cardiovascular disease and osteoporosis for some women
• Improves sleep, particularly if nocturnal hot flashes or night sweats are a problem

The main disadvantages of HRT that have been identified so far are:

- Increases the risk of breast cancer if you take HRT for a long time or take large dosages of estrogen (i.e., greater than .625 mg).
- Side effects like water retention, headaches and rashes.
- Increased chance of yeast infections.
- The combination of estrogen and progestin usually makes women experience return of their monthly periods for several months or longer.

The research on HRT is still not complete, so information on the risks and advantages may change in the next few years. When making the decision to take hormone replacements, get as much information as you can on the risks and benefits for your particular health situation. For example, because of the benefits, women who have severe hot flashes and have family histories of heart disease or osteoporosis are usually advised to go on HRT. However, a family history of breast cancer may make HRT a bad choice for some women. Do not be afraid to get a second opinion from another doctor if you feel your primary physician is not telling you everything or you feel pressured.

Much research, however, indicates that HRT improves sleep for women who have their sleep disrupted by nocturnal hot flashes or other menopause symptoms. Improvements in sleep have been documented in sleep diaries and overnight sleep lab recordings in women taken before and after starting HRT. The main benefit for sleep appears to be the reduced hot flash activity. The daily dosage of estrogen/progestin during menopause seems to help the body regulate temperature better, similar to what a thermostat does in a house. With fewer hot flashes, many women find their sleep improves.

Although there are clear benefits of HRT for sleep, having insomnia during menopause should not be the only reason to start HRT. You need to weigh *all* the advantages and disadvantages of HRT. You may find that by following the :60 Second tips and other strategies provided in this book, you are able to cope with your sleep problems without having to rely on medication. Certainly, if you had

insomnia for many years before you began menopause, you will probably find that HRT will be of limited usefulness in helping you sleep
better. If you have been a chronic insomniac for years and years,
behavior changes and stress management are probably going to do
more for your sleep pattern than most medications, including HRT.

:60 Second Tips for Coping with Menopause-Related Sleep Problems

1. Wear a cotton nightgown or T-shirt to bed. Cotton breathes when
    you sweat, so the moisture does not stay trapped between the fab-
    ric and your skin. You are more likely to cool down wearing cot-
    ton compared to silk, satin or nylon fabrics.
2. Use layers of sheets and cotton bedding on your bed instead of
    one thick comforter or blanket. When you get hot at night, you
    can cool down by throwing off a single layer instead of your
    entire bedding (which would probably result in you getting very
    cold soon after the flash is over). If you share your bed, use your
    own set of bedding on your side, so when you toss off a layer, you
    don't feel guilty about disturbing your bed partner.
3. Put a fan on and direct it toward your bed throughout the night
    during the period of most frequent night sweats. When you are
    cold, use another sheet or blanket to stay warm rather than turn-
    ing the fan off.
4. Take a warm shower or bath right before you go to bed. This will
    keep you cool for the first part of the night. Remember that the
    first half of the night is the time you get most of your deep sleep.
5. Make sure you have things to do when you can't sleep. Recall from
    chapter 7 the importance of getting out of bed when you are not
    sleeping. Staying in bed only prolongs your frustration and con-
    tributes to developing an unhealthy mental association between
    your bed and sleeplessness.
6. Practice these good sleep habits even if you do take HRT.
    Research has actually shown that HRT in combination with a
    behavioral treatment program is more effective against insomnia
    than HRT alone.[3]

If you never had serious sleep problems before menopause, the nocturnal disturbances (that is, hot flashes and night sweats) that come with menopause can be very stressful. It is important to remind yourself that it is a temporary problem that will eventually get better. Most women experience night to night variations, with lots of good nights of sleep in between the bad nights. For many, the severe hot flashes only last a short period of time. While this is going on, try to practice good sleep habits and avoid giving in to the bad ones, even if they give you temporary relief. You don't want a short-term sleep problem becoming a chronic one because of poor insomnia coping skills. Here is a suggested list of other dos and don'ts:

- Never use alcohol to help you sleep.
- Be cautious in how much you nap. A long nap during the day will make your sleep lighter at night, leaving you more susceptible to being awakened at night from hot flashes or night sweats.
- Avoid the temptation to use sleeping pills. Many people who start using sleeping pills for a short-term sleep problem find they end up relying on them for much longer than they intended.

Other Sleep Concerns of Women

Although most sleep disorders occur in men and women in roughly equal numbers, the exception to this is sleep apnea, which is eight times more common in men than women. Pre-menopausal women in particular seem to be protected from sleep apnea. After menopause, however, the rate of sleep apnea increases sharply in women. The risk factors for men and women are the same: obesity, smoking and loud snoring. Among women who do show signs of interrupted breathing at night, the overall severity is generally less than men and the daytime consequences are not as profound. For example, the extreme daytime sleepiness that usually accompanies sleep apnea does not appear to be as severe in women. Although this sounds good, it also means that many women have sleep apnea but are not aware of it. Hence, it goes untreated.

There may be a physiological basis for pre-menopausal women being protected against sleep apnea. The hormone progesterone stimulates breathing in both women and men when they are given the hormone in pill form. After menopause, progesterone levels drop and the protection against sleep apnea may be lost. Although this rationale makes sense, it may not be that simple after all. The risk of sleep apnea increases with age, so women may be more susceptible for reasons other than hormone changes. For example, weight gain in women after menopause is common and research has shown that weight and age are better predictors of sleep apnea in women than hormone levels. Furthermore, a research study showed that giving progestin (the pill form of naturally occurring progesterone) to postmenopausal women resulted in little improvement in obstructive sleep apnea.[4] It would appear for now that the best treatment for sleep apnea in women is the same as men: weight loss, quitting smoking and, in more severe cases, surgery to remove the obstruction or utilizing the continuous positive airway pressure (C-PAP) system.

Whether a woman experiencing sleep problems is in her childbearing years, pre-menopausal or post-menopausal, utilizing the :60 Second tips and recommendations in this book will help her achieve the restorative sleep she seeks. While hormone replacement therapy can help menopausal women specifically with night sweats and hot flashes, acquiring a repertoire of sleep savvy skills and behaviors will provide long-term, lasting sleep improvement.

chapter 13

CHILDREN AND ADOLESCENTS

In this chapter you will:
- *Learn about normal sleep and common sleep disorders in children*
- *Find out why teenagers seem to need so much sleep*
- *Learn tips for coping with your teenager's sleep habits*

Sleep problems are not unique to adults. Many children, including infants, can have problems sleeping. Recent surveys indicate that about 25 percent of children ages one to five experience some form of sleep disturbance. The sleep problems of most children are not severe enough to seek professional help and usually go away on their own or with a little help from the parents. However, disturbed sleep is still one of the most common reasons parents seek help from mental health professionals for their children. In one survey of parents who were referred to child psychiatrists for consultations regarding the sleep problems of their children, the most common problems were talking during sleep (32 percent), nightmares (31 percent), waking through the night (28 percent), trouble falling asleep (23 percent), bed-wetting (17 percent), teeth grinding (10 percent) and night terrors (7 percent). Many children had more than one kind of sleep problem.[1]

Not all children with sleep problems have sleep disorders. Learning to sleep through the night is a developmental milestone that many children and parents struggle with during the children's early years. Waking up throughout the night is not a disorder, but a common sleep behavior. In many cases, parents can help train their children to sleep through the night by letting them fall asleep on their own and resisting the urge to respond immediately to their nighttime stirrings. Having nightmares is another common occurrence in young children that in most cases is not a disorder. Both of these are examples of sleep behaviors and not all behaviors are disorders.

Attaching diagnostic labels to children, while often justified, can also do more harm than good. Labels may cause children to feel that they are to blame for the problem or that they are defective or abnormal. Therefore, resist assigning labels; do not immediately assume your child has a sleep disorder. Children's sleep problems are usually caused by the same type of temporary environmental stressors that disrupt adults' sleep. Children, however, are often unable to verbalize what is bothering them. Thus, parents need to do some detective work to determine the sources of stress for their children. The following table lists a number of useful questions to ask yourself when your child starts to have sleep problems:

Have there been any changes in your family recently?
Examples of change:
- Sibling or other family member has moved out of the home
- Arrival of a new baby
- Death of a family pet
- Death of a grandparent or other close relative
- Moving
- Divorce

Has there been an increase in tension or conflict between you and your spouse lately? Children become very anxious when their parents are not getting along. Many parents attempt to shield their children from their marital problems, however, this can make some kids more anxious, because they know something is wrong, but no one is talking about it.

How is your son or daughter doing at school or in day care?
- A conflict between your child and one or more other children may manifest as trouble sleeping or nightmares. Children are often

embarrassed to tell their parents about problems with other kids, because they fear they may get blamed or looked down upon.

- Falling behind the other kids in school may be caused by something simple like a visual or hearing impairment. Some learning disabilities are actually caused by undetected vision or auditory problems.

Does your small child seem depressed? When children get depressed it often goes unnoticed. Sometimes young children do not have the verbal skills to say, "I'm depressed, Mom."

Some of the signs of depression in children are:

- Seems withdrawn (spends a lot of time in room alone) or the opposite, he or she is very clingy to parents (never wants to be alone)
- Cries more often, sometimes for no reason
- Seems more irritable or angry than usual
- Has a poor appetite
- Regresses in things like toilet training (starts to wet or soil self again)
- Trouble concentrating and more forgetful than usual

How are your child's eating habits? A change in diet can affect sleep patterns. Parents are not always aware of everything their children eat during the day. Ask your child about snacks between meals, particularly foods containing caffeine or other stimulants (e.g., chocolate).

- Some food allergies (cow's milk, for example) can cause mild symptoms like indigestion, bloating, cramps and abdominal gas, all of which can disturb sleep. Check for any new foods or beverages your child has started to consume.
- In addition, make sure your child is not going to bed hungry. If there is a large time period between dinner and bedtime, a light snack before sleep will ensure he or she is not waking up because of hunger.

Normal Developmental Changes in Sleep
Infants
First three months. Newborn babies sleep as much as sixteen hours a day. Of course, they don't sleep all of these hours in a row but usually in two to three hour stretches. They also alternate between periods of

sleep and wakefulness throughout the day *and* night (much to the cha-
grin of mom and dad). Infants get lots of REM and deep sleep, much
more than older children and adults, and they also have shorter sleep
cycles. In chapter 3 we discussed the fact that adults cycle through the
five sleep stages (that is, stages one to four and REM sleep) about every
ninety minutes or so. For new babies, the sleep cycle is about fifty minutes, but this gradually gets longer as they age. It is normal for babies
to wake up two to three times a night from birth until six months. From
six to twelve months old, babies wake up about once or twice per night.
Babies who previously had colic and premature babies may take a little
longer until their sleep patterns are more continuous.

       During the first three months of an infant's life the normal
cues for wake and sleep, namely the rising and setting of the sun, do
not really mean much to him or her. Infants basically go through periods of wakefulness and sleep around the clock without schedules. As
most parents will attest, babies usually wake up hungry and signal
their desire with loud cries directed toward their moms. New mothers
frequently find themselves nursing around the clock. As babies grow,
their stomachs get bigger and they can eat more food at once. The
interval between feedings gets longer and they start to sleep for longer
periods. However, parents need to be cautious about overfeeding
babies at night. Drinking a lot of milk leads to a large production of
urine and a very full bladder. An over distended bladder can awaken a
baby from sleep. In addition, excessive urination results in a very wet
and heavy diaper which may make sleep uncomfortable for baby.

       Three to six months of age. By the age of three months,
babies are generally sleeping for longer periods and beginning to do
more sleeping at night versus the daytime. Most babies will be awake
for longer periods during the day, usually taking two to three long
naps. During these months, he or she is becoming more social and
wants to stay awake longer to play and get attention from mom and
dad. He or she may need to be encouraged to nap—missing one is
likely to result in baby becoming overtired and irritable.

       By the age of six months, all infants have the ability to sleep
through the night. Their stomachs are big enough so that they should
not get hungry during the night. Furthermore, they have sleep cycles

that closely resemble adults' cycles. However, not all babies sleep through the night by six months of age, as many parents will attest. Both sleep and baby experts agree that the achievement of continuous nighttime sleeping is largely a product of how parents respond to their children's nighttime cries from about four months of age and on. Parents seem to follow one of two paths. The most common advice to parents is to let babies older than four months cry until they fall back to sleep on their own.[2] The only times you would not do this is if the child is sick or shows signs of extreme distress. Remember that it is normal for everyone to reach a waking state during the night. Older children and adults can fall back to sleep on their own (unless they suffer from insomnia), a skill that babies also have to learn. Other parents, however, find it very hard to let their children cry at night and continue to respond to children's cries until they are much older than six months.

Ultimately, it is a matter of personal choice for parents. However, be prepared to get up several times a night if you cannot tolerate your baby crying. If you do decide to get up when your baby cries, you should try not to remove him from his sleeping place. Try soothing words or a song while he is lying in the crib or place your hand gently on his to provide additional comfort. Do this until baby falls back asleep. Over time, gradually increase the amount of time before you respond to your baby's crying (for example from five to ten minutes, then ten to twenty minutes gradually and over several nights). Eventually, your baby should start to fall back asleep on his or her own before you even have to get up.

Sudden infant death syndrome. A fear of every new parent is Sudden Infant Death Syndrome (SIDS). Medical experts still don't know what causes SIDS. We do know that it usually occurs during sleep in children under six months old, however, it is not clear if SIDS is a sleep disorder. The chances of SIDS are greater if the infant is allowed to sleep in the facedown (on the stomach) position and when the infant is heavily wrapped in bedding. In the last ten years the incidence of SIDS has dropped quite dramatically as there are significant public health campaigns advising parents to place babies on their backs when sleeping. The rate of SIDS in the United States has decreased by 30 percent; in the United Kingdom a similar campaign has reduced the incidence of SIDS by half!

Preschool Children

As children become older, their sleep patterns get more regular and therefore predictable. Toddlers sleep much less than babies, but still need an average of ten hours a day. Remember that this is only an average and some toddlers get by on much less sleep. As children grow older, their need for daytime naps decreases. Most children no longer need to nap by the time they are four or five; a small percentage of children still need one short nap in the afternoon. Phasing out naps is probably a good practice—a tired child is much easier to get to bed at night. In place of an afternoon nap, many parents and day care centers impose a short period of quiet resting time in the child's afternoon schedule.

Most preschool-age children still get lots of deep sleep at night. Deep sleep is when growth usually occurs, as the pituitary gland secretes human growth hormone. In addition to stimulating growth, human growth hormone helps to maintain and repair the body. For example, broken bones and torn muscles are mostly healed at night while a child sleeps. In addition to physical growth, sleep is a time of mental and emotional growth. Recent studies have suggested that children consolidate their memories during REM sleep. Hence, sleep is important for the acquisition of new knowledge and learning. Research has shown that when older children are given learning tasks and then selectively deprived of REM sleep, they show poor recall of the test items compared to students who are allowed to sleep normally after the task. In other research, brain scans show that the areas of the brain responsible for memories and emotional processing get more blood flow during REM sleep. This process actually continues into adulthood, although childhood is a time when the brain physically grows and new neural connections are formed at an amazing rate. This may explain why infants and young children experience more REM sleep than do adults. Even dreaming may serve an important function in the emotional development of children by helping them adapt to intense emotional states like fear or anger.

:60 Second Tips for Helping Children Sleep Better

- Hold and soothe infants frequently during the day. Physical contact helps them to feel safe and secure in their home and stimulates growth.

- The child's sleeping environment should be quiet, dark (except maybe for a nightlight) and have a constant temperature that is neither too hot or cold. The bedroom should be familiar, comforting and relaxing.

- Having a consistent evening and bedtime routine will help a child get ready for sleep. A relaxing, nurturing presleep routine such as a bath and reading a book will help a child associate sleep with things that are pleasant and comforting.

- Avoid using going to bed early as a form of punishment. Children may come to associate the bed with feeling bad or guilty. Whenever possible, misbehavior in the evening should be punished or corrected in some other way.

- Do not take daytime naps too late in the afternoon and not too long in length. Naps longer than one hour and after 3:00 P.M. will probably interfere with nighttime sleep.

- Keep a consistent bedtime and waking up time throughout the entire week, not just weekdays.

- Give children a light snack and drink before bed. This may help prevent children from going to bed hungry. Refrain from acceding to demands for more drinks, food or stories. This may reinforce the child's avoidance of going to bed.

Sleep Disorders in Children

The most common sleep disorders in children are: (the disorders are arranged from the most common to least common).

Nightmares

It is normal for children to have nightmares. They are very common in children between the ages of four and nine.[3] Hence, the occasional nightmare is to be expected and may even be beneficial to emotionally prepare children for nightmares when they get older. It is not uncommon for a child to have a nightmare after seeing a scary movie or experiencing something upsetting during the day. Major changes in the home (for example, a new baby) may also trigger nightmares. Some children may have recurring nightmares several days in a row and then not have them for a long time. The time to become concerned is when the nightmares become chronic (for example, when they go on nightly for more than a couple of weeks) and disturb your child's sleep enough that she is tired during the day. Younger children will have a harder time understanding their nightmares. Reassure your child that what happens in nightmares is not real. The more you get your child to talk about the nightmare, the more she will realize it was just a dream and she is safe.

Persistent nightmares do not mean that your child is abnormal or mentally ill. In most cases, nightmares relate to something going on in the child's life during the day. The child may be having difficulty adjusting to school, may not be getting along with a playmate or may sense that something is wrong at home. Instability in the home is a common cause of nightmares. The most effective treatment is finding out what is really bothering your child and talking about it openly. In some cases, a recurring nightmare is about a specific fear the child has developed (such as a fear of dogs, snakes, water, falling, etc.) or may be a delayed response to a traumatic event the child experienced (sudden death of a friend or family member, for example). The nightmare may be a subconscious expression of their anxiety about the feared object or traumatic event. If your child has trouble describing the fear, ask him or her to draw it on a piece of paper and then talk openly about the drawing. Do not be surprised if there is little logic or reason behind the basis of the feared object in younger children (for example, a child who is afraid "dinosaurs live in the garden"). Provide comfort and reassurance and avoid minimizing or discounting your child's fears with statements like, "It's silly to be afraid of that."

With more severe fears, professional counseling may be needed to help the child overcome or cope better with the anxiety. Older children (twelve years and older) may respond to behavioral methods such as systematic desensitization. This is a treatment in which the individual is gradually exposed to the feared object until his or her anxiety reaction lessens and then eventually dissipates. The approach is very successful in helping people conquer their fears.

Sleepwalking

About 15 percent of all children will have at least one episode of sleepwalking. For about 3 percent of children, it becomes a chronic problem. Contrary to the name, not all kids actually walk—some just sit up in their bed and appear to be awake. Many children sleepwalk and sleep talk at the same time, although what the child says (or mumbles) is often incomprehensible, because they articulate poorly or speak the words out of sequence. Full episodes of sleepwalking last about ten minutes. The child may get out of bed and walk about the house doing ordinary things like getting dressed, going to the bathroom (though not always in the toilet!) and may even attempt to leave the house. Typically, the child returns to bed and has no memory of the incident in the morning.

The phenomenon of sleepwalking is an excellent illustration of the mysterious nature of sleep. Sleepwalking usually occurs when the individual is in deep (slow-wave) sleep. Normally, a person in deep sleep is completely relaxed and lying immobile in bed. The brain is at its quietest point during the night in deep sleep, making this stage of sleep the most restorative. Therefore, it is ironic that sleepwalking occurs at this point of the sleep cycle. In fact, sleepwalking tends to occur during the last part of a period of deep sleep, just when the sleeper is about to shift into a lighter stage of sleep. This is why sleepwalking is considered an arousal disorder. In between sleep stages, the brain may get confused and prematurely signal the body that an awakening is coming soon. An episode of sleepwalking may be a partial arousal—the body seems awake, but the brain is fast asleep. Children are more likely to sleepwalk than adults simply because they have more deep sleep and also because their brains are still developing (the brain of a child is more likely to have these partial arousals when sleep and wake get confused).

Sleepwalking usually starts between the ages of four and eight and peaks at about twelve years of age. The course of the disorder is usually irregular—the child may sleepwalk several nights in a row and then sleep normally for months afterward. Episodes may be brought on by stress, high fever or excitement (before a birthday party, for example), but they often occur for no apparent reason. Most children who sleepwalk are otherwise healthy and emotionally well-adjusted. Since there is no standard treatment for sleepwalking, the best thing parents can do is to safety proof the house and make sure the doors are securely locked at night. Limit the amount of liquids consumed in the evening and encourage your child to empty his bladder right before bedtime—this will prevent any "accidents" from occurring during one of his nocturnal walks. It is best not to wake a sleepwalker unless he or she is about to go outside or do something that may cause injury. Sleepwalking children can usually be guided back to bed and tucked in without waking them up. You can do this by lightly touching your child on the shoulder and speaking quietly and calmly.

Bed-wetting

Bed-wetting is very common. After toilet training is finished, usually by the time the child is three years old, occasional "accidents" during sleep are to be expected. In fact, about 30 percent of four-year-olds wet the bed at least once and typically several times. Such episodes are not really a sleep disorder because it usually takes some time for children to achieve full bladder control. Persistent bed-wetting after the age of five is the core symptom for sleep *enuresis*, which is the medical term for bed-wetting. About 10 percent of six-year olds and 5 percent of ten-year olds are persistent bed wetters. A small number of children are spontaneously cured, meaning that the condition goes away on its own.

The cause of bed-wetting is still not fully understood. There may be a genetic factor, because children who wet the bed are more likely than other children to have a parent who also had the problem as a child. There may also be a gender factor, because the condition is more common in boys than girls. For about 5 percent to 10 percent of children there is a definite medical cause to bed-wetting such as a bladder infection or diabetes. If your child starts to suddenly wet the bed after a long period of good bladder control, it is wise to take him or her to the doctor to ensure there is not a physical cause. It is believed that anxiety and emotional distress can precipitate enuresis for some children. In general, the older the child, the more likely the cause of bed-wetting is a health problem or an emotionally stressful event.

For most children, bed-wetting seems to start for no apparent reason. The onset of bed-wetting is likely to bring on anxiety in the child about going to bed. Hence, children have their sleep disturbed by two sources, the wetness and discomfort associated with the accident and the fear of going to sleep. Children often feel shame and embarrassment about the problem and may start avoiding social outings like sleepovers or camping with friends. If left untreated, bed-wetting can be quite damaging to the child's self-esteem and social development.

The good news is that bed-wetting is highly treatable. The most effective method is the bell and pad system with a success rate of 80 percent. With this system, a bell sounds as soon as the pad detects moisture, waking up the child so he can go and urinate in the toilet. Other treatment approaches include medication, hypnosis and counseling. Parents are advised to continually reassure the child that they do not believe he or she is wetting the bed on purpose and to provide hope that the problem will be resolved. Parents should restrict evening beverages and encourage the child to empty his or her bladder before going to bed. Scolding or punishing your child for bed-wetting is likely to make him or her feel more tense and helpless, which will likely only make the problem worse.

Night Terrors

Although they have similar names, nightmares and night terrors are actually very different sleep disorders. After a child wakes up from a nightmare, he usually remembers the content of his dream. In contrast, a child does not associate night terrors with a scary dream. In fact, many children are not aware they have night terrors. Night terrors actually have more in common with sleepwalking. With both disorders, the events in question happen during deep sleep (compared to nightmares, which occur mostly during REM sleep) and children usually have no memory of the events in the morning. Night terrors will cause the child to scream at night, usually loud enough to waken the rest of the house. He may stare into space for a minute or two, appearing terrified but often will not wake up. If left alone, the child will usually return to a resting sleep state. Sometimes, the child will jump out of bed and rush about the room frantically until he wakes up. However, it is dangerous to attempt to restrain the child while this is happening. It is better to make the room injury-proof (for example, put padding on sharp corners of furniture, keep the floor clear of toys so the child will not trip and fall) and wait for the child to return to bed or wake up on his or her own.

Night terrors are usually more distressing to parents than to children. They are rare, occurring in only about 3 percent of all children and are most common in older male children. Night terrors are often resolved on their own usually by the time of adolescence. For extreme cases in which there is a risk of injury, benzodiazepine medication may be used to suppress deep sleep. Unlike nightmares, there is no solid evidence that night terrors are related to daytime fears, environmental stressors or emotional disturbances. Night terrors tend to run in families, so there is a possibility that they are due in part to genetic factors.

Teeth Grinding

Bruxism is the grinding or clenching of the teeth during sleep. Over half of healthy infants grind their teeth at night as their primary teeth start to grow in and their little mouths get used to these new protrusions. Most children adapt to their new teeth and only grind them occasionally. Chronic bruxism, on the other hand, can cause dental problems like abnormal wearing down of the teeth, headaches and persistent jaw pain. Available statistics suggest that chronic bruxism is a rare condition. When it does occur, it usually starts between the ages of ten and twenty years old. Like many sleep disorders, stress is thought to be a precipitating factor. Treatment approaches range from wearing a nighttime tooth guard (a rubber or plastic prosthetic molded to the shape of the individual's teeth) to stress management and biofeedback. There is not much information on effective treatments for children. If you suspect your child has chronic bruxism, discuss the situation with your physician or dentist to explore treatment options.

Sleep Apnea

We discussed sleep apnea in chapter 2. It occurs mostly in adults, but can also appear in children. Snoring is the main symptom, but snoring alone is not enough to confirm a child has apnea. Only about one in five children who snore actually have obstructive sleep apnea. Other signs of sleep apnea in children include:

- Extreme sleepiness during the day
- Difficulty breathing during sleep
- Daytime breathing through the mouth instead of the nose
- Labored swallowing
- Sleeping in odd positions
- Sweating during sleep

The disorder is more common in boys than girls. Diagnosis is usually made when the child is around seven years old, although many children have the disorder for quite some time before getting diagnosed. Children who are extremely overweight are most at risk to develop sleep apnea.

The most common form of treatment is surgery to clear the airway. For 70 percent of children, removing the tonsils or adenoids is followed by a sharp decrease in symptoms. If left untreated, sleep apnea can delay intellectual growth, language development and performance in school.

Medications for Children

Treatment for sleep disorders in children generally consists of parental reassurance and comfort, behavior modification techniques and, in some cases, counseling for the child. Giving children medications specifically for sleep problems is discouraged for a variety of reasons. Like adults, most sleep medications provide only a temporary solution and often do not address the underlying causes of the sleep problems. Furthermore, children are even more susceptible to the side effects of medications. On a more fundamental level, most sleep problems in children are part of the normal developmental changes that children experience and medicating them away does not give your child the opportunity to adapt and cope in more natural ways. If your doctor suggests a medication for your child's sleep difficulties, you should seriously question the benefits and ask about all the side effects. Find out if a non-drug, alternative therapy is available. The exception to this would be cases in which a medical condition is the root cause of your child's sleep problems (for example, a bladder infection that causes nighttime incontinence). In this situation, medication would be quite appropriate.

Medications to treat other medical conditions may also cause sleep disturbances. Some drugs have stimulating effects and can frequently disrupt sleep. An example of this is the medication Ritalin, which is used to treat attention deficit and hyperactivity disorder (ADHD). Ritalin is a powerful stimulant and insomnia is the most common side effect. You can limit the impact of Ritalin on sleep by ensuring that the last dosage your child takes during the day is at least four hours before bedtime. Insomnia is a side effect of many other medications including nasal decongestants, corticosteroids and bronchodilators (puffers) used for asthma. Common pain medications such as aspirin can reduce deep sleep, making your child's sleep shallower and less refreshing. In most cases, sleep disturbances associated with drug use are short-lived and only last as long as your child needs to take the medication.

Adolescents and Sleep

Among the many conflicts between parents and teenagers, sleep habits seem to rank among the most common for the majority of parents that we interview. The biggest complaints about teens and sleep seem to be:

- He is unable to get up at the same time as the rest of the house; and always seem to be in a rush or late to get to school
- She wants to stay up past midnight every night despite having school the next day
- He stays out very late on weekends and then sleeps in past noon
- Despite spending so much time in bed, she seems to be tired all the time

Fortunately, researchers have started to listen to the concerns of parents and their teenage sons and daughters in the last fifteen years and we are starting to have a better understanding of adolescent sleep patterns and sleep needs. Furthermore, we are starting to see that there is a high percentage of sleep disorders in teenagers. Many are, in fact, sleep deprived and their daytime performance in school and everyday activities like driving may be affected. The challenge for parents is to sort out what seems to be legitimate sleep problems in their teens from what the parents may see as defiant or uncooperative behaviors.

Do Teenagers Need More Sleep?

Teenagers are still children and their sleep needs don't change that much from pre-teenage life to adolescence. The average teen needs about eight and one-half to nine and one-half hours of sleep a night. For parents who only need to sleep six and one-half to seven and one-half hours a night, sleeping nine hours at night seems like a marathon. Nevertheless, most teenagers don't get anywhere near the amount of sleep they need on typical nights. Staying up past midnight and then getting up for school at 7:00 A.M. or so means your son or daughter only gets about 80 percent of the sleep they need from Sunday to Thursday. During the week they accumulate a "sleep debt" that they typically attempt to recover on the weekend.

Consider that the average teen needs sixty-three hours of sleep a week (average of nine hours per night times seven nights per week) but only sleeps seven hours a night from Sunday to Thursday. This means that he or she has slept thirty-five hours by the time Friday rolls around and needs to recover ten hours of lost sleep sometime on the weekend, in addition to the usual nine hours a night they should be getting. That is fourteen hours of sleep a night for Friday and Saturday! Fortunately, most teens do not sleep fourteen hours in a row on weekend nights. This is because most people can recover a sleep debt in less time than it was incurred. You will recall from chapter 2 that people who are sleep deprived can recover the all important REM and deep sleep in less time than usual on recovery times. Nevertheless, a teen wanting to sleep ten to twelve hours a night on the weekend makes sense once you have done the math.

For many teens their bedrooms are also their sanctuaries and their desire to spend long hours there is not motivated solely by a need for sleep. They may simply like the privacy of their bedroom and, in particular, time away from other family members and obligations like school and chores. Consequently, they may fiercely protect their Saturday mornings for sleeping, resting, listening to music or whatever suits them. Similarly, these teenagers may view late evenings after the rest of the family has gone to bed as the same sort of protected time.

Delayed Sleep Phase Syndrome

Much has been written lately on adolescents having internal clocks that are out of sync with the rest of the adult world. Teens go to bed later each year they get older. The average eighteen-year-old's bedtime is past midnight. Studies of high school students have shown that their natural bed times are 11:00 P.M. or later. Many adults also make this their bedtime, but their sleep needs are different from a child. A teenager who needs nine hours of sleep at night would have to wake up at 8:00 A.M. or later, which doesn't leave much time to prepare for school (particularly if school starts at 8:00A.M.!).

There may be a biological basis for this kind of sleep pattern in teens. Scientists who have studied the circadian timing system of adolescents have concluded that they have internal clocks that are delayed one to two hours compared to adults. One of the signs of this delay is the secretion of melatonin by the pineal gland. Melatonin is an important hormone involved in helping the body maintain a twenty-four-hour cycle. It is only produced after dark and peak production occurs in the middle of the night; thus, the level of melatonin in the body is lowest during the day. Higher levels of melatonin are a biological signal to the brain to begin nighttime behavior. In adolescents, melatonin levels peak later than adults. Hence, their brains don't get the signal to begin sleep until later in the evening. Using the analogy of time zones, it is as if teenagers go by an internal clock that is set *one to two time zones to the west* of their parents. So, if you are living in Eastern Standard Time, your son or daughter may be on Central or Mountain Time. In other words, they are not ready to go to bed until one or two hours (or more) after their parents. This is referred to as *delayed sleep phase syndrome* (DSPS).

Researchers who study DSPS have not figured out what causes it. One of the questions being asked is whether adolescents develop this delayed sleep pattern naturally (meaning it could be genetic or bio-logically determined in some way) or whether it comes about because of lifestyle and environmental factors. In reality, it is probably a bit of both. Some of the psychological and lifestyle influences on DSPS could be:

- Many teenagers push the limits of their daytime activities. A typical day can consist of being at school by 8:30 A.M. or earlier, attending school all day, perhaps one to two hours of sports practice after school, getting home and having dinner, one to two hours of homework, phone calls to friends planning their busy social life, watching television and, finally, bed by 12:30 or 1:00 A.M.
- On weekends, teens like to stay out late to be with their friends no matter how tired they may be feeling. They like to push the limits of weekend outings, perhaps out of some minor rebellion, but also the desire to be out with their friends for as long as possible (how many times has your teenager come home earlier than his or her appointed curfew?).
- Entertainment that attracts teens seem to start later in the evenings. The best television shows (from a teen's perspective) are on late, movies in the theaters play at all hours, many teen dances don't start until late and are planned so that they last virtually all night ("raves," for example) and, of course, the always available Internet.
- Adolescence is a time of both physical and emotional stress. Many teenagers have lots of worries: dating, getting high grades, main-taining a social life, doing well in sports, etc. Stress and worrying tend to delay sleep onset in both adolescents and adults.
- Lots of parents stay up late watching television or doing other things. A teenager may be emulating his mom and dad. Unfortunately, the sleep needs of mom and dad are quite differ-ent from their teen's.

In light of DSPS, many sleep experts are advocating that high school boards restructure the school schedule to accommodate the sleep patterns and sleep needs of teenagers. They argue that the cur-rent start time of 8:00 to 8:30 A.M. in most schools is too early for teenagers. Some schools start even earlier. The consequence of such an early start time is that kids begin their day feeling tired and unmotivated to learn. Furthermore, having arisen late, many are in such a rush in the morning that breakfast is often skipped. By starting an hour later, teenagers would be more alert and able to process new learning. School boards appear to be taking this advice seriously, because some have changed to later school start times. There are examples of schools in the United States in which later start times have resulted in a number of improvements in students, including sleeping more hours, better moods, increased grades and more time for extracurricular activities.[4] On the other hand, some schools found that the shift to a later start time caused additional problems such as schedule conflicts with after school jobs and extracurricular activities.

We should also point out that not all teenagers have the problem known as DSPS. Many teens have no bigger problem getting up at 7:00 A.M. for school than do adults who have to get up for work. Furthermore, DSPS seems to be largely a problem of urban teens. Children who grow up in farm communities generally are quite used to going to bed early and getting up much earlier than their city counterparts. For teens in rural areas, there are fewer environmental temptations to stay up late and sleep in on the weekends.

Insomnia in Teens

Several years ago the National Institutes of Health concluded adolescents were a high risk group for developing serious sleep problems. This initiated a study of sleep in teens, conducted by the National Sleep Foundation (NSF). It was published in 1997 and is available online from their Web site at www.sleepfoundation.org.[5] Teenagers who complain of insomnia are often dismissed by their parents and teachers with statements like, "You wouldn't be so tired if you went to bed earlier" or "It's your own fault for staying out so late on the weekends." Granted, many of the sleep problems in teenagers start because of poor sleep habits, but then again so do the sleep problems of most adults. Teenagers have just as much stress as adults, maybe even more, because they often do not have the emotional maturity to manage stress effectively. A relatively small problem—not having a date for the spring dance—can be seen as a major crisis in the mind of teenager, one that can bother her for days or weeks at a time.

The rate of insomnia in adolescents is about 14 percent, which is lower than adults, but still translates into millions of teens who do not feel they are getting enough sleep. The pattern of insomnia in teenagers is different than in adults. The symptoms (difficulty falling asleep is usually the main one) typically are shorter in duration and more irregular. For example, a teen may have poor sleep during the week but then have a sleep "marathon" on the weekend to catch up on lost sleep. She may sleep fine for a couple of weeks until it starts over again. The cause of insomnia in teens is most often stress-related. Most teens have not developed the conditioned insomnia pattern typically seen in adult insomniacs, because most teens still get stretches of good sleep. However, many adult insomniacs report that their sleep problems began during adolescence and got progressively worse over time. It is possible that many cases of adult insomnia could have been prevented by developing good sleep habits as teens, when they were most vulnerable to develop bad ones.

In addition to stress, insomnia in adolescents is often related to poor health practices. Teenagers who smoke, for example, are more likely to have insomnia. Like adults, many teens smoke as a way of coping with stress. However, the nicotine in cigarettes has the opposite effect because it makes you tense and agitated instead of relaxed. Alcohol use in teens can also cause sleep problems. Teenage consumption of alcohol typically resembles binge drinking patterns. They may not drink any alcohol during the week and then drink large quantities on the weekend. You may recall from chapter 2 that alcohol negatively affects sleep by reducing the amount of deep sleep and causing more awakenings as the body goes through alcohol withdrawal. Teenagers who binge drink on the weekend are likely to spend many hours in bed "sleeping it off." However, the sleep they do get is of extremely poor quality, leading them to wake up feeling even more tired and groggy.

There are many possible consequences of poor sleep for adolescents. Studies have shown that high school students who report having academic problems also report getting less sleep and having more irregular sleep schedules compared to students who get higher grades. As with adults, poor sleep seems to go along with symptoms of depression, anxiety and also impulse control problems and mood swings. Students who report having poor sleep are more likely to use stimulant types of drugs (caffeine and nicotine) and consume more alcohol.

Another serious problem is teens driving when they are sleep deprived. Teenagers and young adults are already over represented in the statistics on traffic fatalities. Many traffic crashes are the results of falling asleep at the wheel. Data collected in the state of North Carolina revealed that over half of the motor vehicles involved in fall-asleep crashes were driven by people twenty-five years of age and under.[6] Car accidents are still the leading cause of death for people between the ages of fifteen and twenty. Most traffic fatalities with young adults involve alcohol and many occur after midnight. The combination of alcohol, sleep deprivation, driving late at night and driver inexperience can be, to say the least, deadly for young persons and those they encounter on the road.

:60 Second Sleep Tips for Parents of Teenagers
1.   Avoid arguing over the issue of staying up late and sleeping in. In most cases, arguing is counterproductive and may actually encourage your teenager to do the opposite of what you request.
2.   Do not "reward" teenagers who sleep late on school days and miss their bus with a drive to school. It you do this, be prepared to do it more and more in the future. Encourage your teenager to take responsibility for getting up and getting to school on time.
3.   Allow your teenager to set his or her bedtime. Most teens will resent having set bedtimes because this makes them feel like children. However, set limits on late night activities. Impose strict rules regarding watching television (for example, no television after 10:00 P.M.), using the computer or accepting phone calls after a certain hour. Your teenager can stay up late, but must engage in quiet, relaxing activities such as reading or listening to music.
4.   Set an example for your teenager by following these rules yourself. That is, turn off the television for everyone in the family at 10:00 P.M. (or whatever time you set). Avoid sending your children

"mixed messages" by having a different set of sleep rules for you and your kids.

5. Do not allow your teenager to have a television or computer in his or her room. Ideally, your teen should have another area in the home to complete homework, but this may not be very practical. At a minimum, actively discourage your son or daughter from doing homework on the bed. This may build an association between the bed (which should only be used for sleeping) and an unpleasant activity like homework.

6. Be a role model for your teenager by avoiding caffeinated drinks, alcohol and junk food in the evening.

7. Be flexible about the time that teenagers have to get their chores done on the weekend. Insisting that chores must be done early Saturday morning may not work well with the teenager who likes and may need to sleep in on this day. Negotiate with your son or daughter a time at which chores need to be completed (3:00 P.M. for example), before they can go off to do their own activities.

8. Establish some small rewards to entice your teenager to get up early, a nice breakfast for example. A teenager is not going to be too motivated to get up early on Saturday if the first thing he or she is expected to do upon arising is mow the lawn or clean the garage.

PART 5

LIFESTYLE CHANGES
AND MAINTAINING YOUR PROGRESS

chapter 14

SLEEP HYGIENE: LIFESTYLE CHANGES THAT CAN HELP YOU SLEEP BETTER

In this chapter you will learn:
- *The effects of caffeine and smoking on your sleep*
- *Tips for eating right and how to exercise to promote better sleep*
- *How to create the ideal bedroom environment*

What is Sleep Hygiene?

The term "sleep hygiene" may be unfamiliar to you. When people hear the word "hygiene" they usually think of personal grooming habits or dental hygiene. Actually, "sleep hygiene" refers to a whole group of health, lifestyle and environmental factors that can directly or indirectly affect the amount and quality of sleep you obtain. The goals of this chapter are to increase your awareness of how sleep hygiene can influence your sleep and to provide you with some realistic guidelines on how to change these lifestyle practices and habits that may be harming your sleep. In chapter 2, you learned about the effects of alcohol on sleep and advantages of maintaining abstinence for improving your sleep. In this chapter, you will learn about the impact of caffeine, nicotine, exercise and diet on your sleep.

Sleep hygiene is an integral part of the :60 Second program. Although it is rare that a person's insomnia is caused purely by lifestyle factors, it is often the case that sleep disturbances can be made worse by engaging in one or more negative health behaviors. Such behaviors can slow down a person's progress in a self-management sleep program by exacerbating problems and not allowing their sleep to improve as much as it could. In most cases, the behavioral strategies introduced in previous chapters can be enhanced by changing other lifestyle behaviors.

Lifestyle changes are always a matter of making choices. We recognize that making the decision to eliminate certain health behaviors (smoking, for example) is a big one. For now, we only ask that you at least attempt to modify lifestyle practices for a trial period and examine the effect it has on your sleep. Ideally, the trial period should be at least one month to allow for any withdrawal effects (for example when quitting or reducing smoking or caffeine consumption) to subside and to allow for the transition into new health practices. If at the end of the trial period, you decide you want to maintain these new lifestyle changes, you should consider some additional assistance to keep from returning to your old habits and instead help make the changes permanent.

Caffeine and Sleep

Most people believe caffeine is a relatively harmless substance. North Americans ingest an average of 200 mg of caffeine (approximately two and one-half cups of coffee) per day, primarily in the form of caffeinated beverages such as coffee, tea and cola drinks. With coffee and tea, the stronger it is brewed, the higher the caffeine content. However, many people are not aware that caffeine is present in many other beverages and foods. Although the amount of caffeine in these products varies, the following are average amounts:

- Cup (5 oz.) of brewed coffee = 85 mg caffeine (average)
- Cup (5 oz.) of instant coffee = 65 mg caffeine
- Cup (5 oz.) of brewed tea = 40 mg caffeine
- Hot chocolate (5 oz.) = 6 mg caffeine
- Baker's chocolate (1 oz.) = 26 mg caffeine
- Cola drinks (12 oz.) = 45 mg caffeine

The effects of caffeine on sleep are well-known. Caffeine is a stimulant that acts to excite the central nervous system, leading one to feel more alert and awake. Caffeine disturbs sleep by increasing the amount of time it takes to fall asleep and by decreasing total sleep time. Individuals with chronic sleep difficulties may be even more sensitive than others to the stimulating effects of caffeine. Some people will claim they can drink coffee right up until bedtime and it doesn't affect their sleep. Such individuals are rare. For the majority of people, caffeine affects sleep. This is why it is important to watch your consumption of coffee and other caffeine-laden products.

Even one cup of coffee, tea or cola in the evening is sufficient to disrupt the normal sleeping process. It takes, on average, between three to seven hours for caffeine to be eliminated from the body. This means that the caffeine from a cup of coffee consumed after dinner at 7 P.M. can still be working in your body when you go to bed at 11:00 P.M. Some research suggests that insomniacs take longer to eliminate caffeine from their bodies.[1] This is why it is recommended that you not take any caffeinated food or beverage item after 6:00 P.M. You should also restrict your coffee consumption during the day to a moderate level (no more than two or three cups of coffee per day) or drink decaffeinated coffee.

Caffeine is also an ingredient in many prescription and non-prescription medications, especially over-the-counter pain medications. The amount of caffeine in each pill is small, but the total amount can add up when you are taking many pills per day. For someone who is not a regular caffeine consumer, this amount of caffeine can have quite a powerful stimulant effect. Caffeine is also a diuretic, which means it makes you urinate more. Thus, taking medication with caffeine as an ingredient before sleeping can lead to being awakened frequently with the urge to go the bathroom. Commonly taken medications that contain caffeine are:
- Tylenol with codeine (#1) = 8 mg caffeine
- Excedrin = 65 mg caffeine
- Midol = 32 mg caffeine
- Dristan Decongestant = 16 mg caffeine
- Dexatrim (diet pills) = 200 mg caffeine

Reducing Caffeine Consumption Safely

Many people with insomnia get into the habit of coping with the fatigue caused by poor sleep by drinking large amounts of coffee or other caffeinated beverages during the day. If you are consuming high quantities of caffeine—more than five cups of coffee per day—you should cut down *gradually*. If you don't, you may suffer caffeine withdrawal effects such as headaches and increased nervousness. To reduce gradually, eliminate one daily cup of coffee every three days or gradually switch one of your daily coffees to a decaffeinated brand. Thus, if you are a regular drinker of six cups of coffee per day and you wish to cut this amount down to three cups per day, you should do it gradually over a one to two week period. Be aware also of the caffeine in other products you are consuming and cut that down as well or slowly eliminate it entirely.

With regard to reducing caffeine-containing medications, you should do so under the supervision of your physician. It is likely that there are equivalent caffeine-free medications.

Smoking and Sleep

Nicotine is another stimulant that can disrupt sleep. In fact, smoking is more detrimental than caffeine for sleep because it can cause respiratory problems, making it difficult to breathe at night. Many smokers claim to use cigarettes as a way of coping with stress. It is a common folly among smokers that a cigarette is relaxing. In fact, the "relaxing" effects of a cigarette are really just the suppression of withdrawal symptoms. Nicotine causes the opposite effect of relaxation in the body by increasing heart rate, blood pressure and stimulation in the brain. Most smokers who quit report that they feel much more relaxed and are better able to handle stress than they did as smokers.

Research studies have demonstrated that people who smoke more than one pack per day have shallower and more disrupted sleep than non-smokers. They take longer to get to sleep and have lower sleep efficiencies. Smokers also tend to awaken during the night craving a cigarette. It is not uncommon for smokers to get up in the middle of the night to smoke.[2]

You should know that the stimulating effects of caffeine and nicotine are additive. Thus, smoking and drinking coffee can be doubly harmful to your sleep. Unfortunately, many people who smoke also tend to drink a lot of coffee. It is also unfortunate that both habits are quite difficult to break, although most people are more successful in reducing coffee consumption than quitting smoking. Trying to quit smoking is a major endeavor. Many people try and fail several times before succeeding. If you are one of those people with many failed attempts, you may consider seeking some professional assistance and using a nicotine patch to cope with withdrawal symptoms.

If, on the other hand, you feel you are not ready to completely quit at this time, you should consider reducing your cigarette consumption for the sake of better sleep hygiene. As an experiment, try eliminating five cigarettes per day for one month and see how it affects your sleep. Try to cut out those cigarettes that are pure habit. For example, lighting up while stuck in traffic or after a meal. You should also refrain from smoking three to four hours before bedtime and consider switching to a brand with less nicotine to cut down on the amount of stimulant getting into your body.

Eating Right and Sleep

"I had the worst nightmare last night! It must have been those two chilidogs I ate." Despite popular myth, there is no scientific evidence linking chilidogs, pepperoni or any other spicy food to nightmares. On the other hand, it is likely that eating any large meal close to bedtime, especially a meal that may be taxing on the digestive system (e.g., chilidogs!), will lead to disruptions in the normal sleep cycle. Eating any large quantity of food will stimulate your digestive system. Regarding nightmares, you are more likely to awaken from a bad dream because of the disruption to your sleep cycle brought on by an overactive digestive system. Since you can only remember dreams that you awaken from, you may associate the bad dream with your poor food choice before bed.

Having a *light* snack before bed may actually promote sleep, especially if you incorporate this habit into your pre-bedtime routine. A light combination of carbohydrates and protein, such as cheese and crackers, is good. However, the sleep-promoting aspects of this snack are likely more psychological than biological. Your pre-bedtime snack can serve as part of your pre-sleep ritual, like brushing your teeth.

Certain vitamins and chemical compounds can have mild sleep-promoting effects. In the case of vitamins and minerals, it is more likely that a deficiency in certain ones will cause sleep disturbances.[3] This is why it is important to eat a well-balanced diet that includes the following:

- Magnesium, 350 mg daily
- Calcium, 800 mg daily
- Vitamin B3 (niacin), 75 mg daily
- Vitamin B12 (also known as the stress vitamin), 2 micrograms daily
- Folic Acid, 2-5 mg daily

You can get these vitamins and minerals by taking a multivitamin tablet every day. You can also get them by eating a balanced diet that includes lots of fruits and vegetables. There is no magic food or diet that will ensure you get all the nutrients you need for optimal health. In general, it is best to eat a variety of foods and not too much of any one. You should eat small frequent meals throughout the day. It is better to eat three to five small meals a day than two big meals (for example, eating a big breakfast, skipping lunch and having a big dinner). Many people with insomnia fall into the habit of eating snack foods or worse, fast foods, because they feel too tired too prepare a balanced meal. By doing this, they are depriving themselves of the important nutrients that help fight stress and promote better sleep. Here are some suggestions for ensuring that you eat healthy foods even when you are tired:

- Have fruits and healthy snacks (raisins, sunflower seeds, for example) readily available when you feel hungry but are too tired to make a meal. Carry at least one piece of fruit with you when you leave the house.
- When you do cook, prepare large quantities so you have ready-made meals leftover. For example, make a large salad that will last for several days.

• Don't go grocery shopping when you are hungry. You may be
   tempted to buy quick snack foods instead of healthier choices.

Exercise and Sleep

There are many health benefits to regular physical activity. Exercise can
serve as a protective factor against the development of chronic illnesses such as heart disease. Physical activity can also be a buffer for
the harmful effects of stress. For example, many people use physical
activity as a method of coping with life stressors (e.g., going for a brisk
walk after having a stressful argument with your spouse or friend).
Research has also shown that people who exercise on a regular basis
are less likely to suffer from the long-term harmful physical and emotional effects of chronic stress. In laboratory situations, physically fit
individuals show less physiological arousal (heart rate, blood pressure
and muscle tension) under conditions of mental stress than people
who don't exercise regularly.

There is considerable research affirming that regular physical
activity has positive effects on sleep. The reasons for this appear to
be related to sleep's function as a restorative mechanism for the body.
In essence, it is thought that the more active a person is, the more
energy he or she will have to recover during sleep. Deep sleep is particularly affected by physical activity. Studies have shown that physically active individuals spend more time in deep sleep than inactive
individuals. They also take less time to fall asleep and have fewer
awakenings. Paradoxically, physically fit persons tend to sleep fewer
hours during the night, probably because their sleep is deeper and less
fragmented.

You don't have to be an athlete to reap the benefits of exercise. In reality, it is more important to engage in *regular* mild to moderate exercise. Walking is a good example of this and an activity that
almost everyone can handle. Heart specialists advise regular walking
as a preventive measure for heart disease. *Irregular* bursts of strenuous exercise frequently do more harm than good. For example, muscle aches and pains from occasional exercise can be painful and this
may scare you off from future exercise. In contrast, most people find
it easy to incorporate a daily walk or perhaps a bicycle ride into their

routine. Here are a few tips for selecting and planning a regular
regime of physical activity:

- Before doing any exercise, do some stretching exercises to loosen
  up stiff muscles—this will help to reduce any aches or discomfort
  that may occur during the activity or afterwards.
- Find activities to do in a group or with a friend. Here are some
  examples: walking, swimming, cycling, dancing. Having someone to
  share the experience with can make it more enjoyable and something
  to look forward to. You can also give each other support and praise.
- DON'T do any heavy exercise just before bedtime. The increased
  arousal (elevated heart rate, blood pressure and body temperature)
  can disrupt your ability to get to sleep. The best time to exercise
  is in the morning or late afternoon before 6:00 P.M.
- Plan a mild, pleasurable activity, such as walking, for first thing
  when you get up in the morning; this will give you an incentive for
  arising at a regular hour.
- Choose an activity that you can do on a regular basis regardless of
  the season. Again, walking is the prime example. It can be done in
  virtually any weather condition. Also, you can always find ways of
  making it interesting (e.g., walk with a new friend, change your route).

Best Sleeping Environment

Room temperature can affect how well you sleep. For example, most
people find it difficult to sleep in a really warm room. Hot summer
nights can be terrible for sleeping, especially if you already experience
poor sleep. High temperatures (above approximately eighty degrees
Fahrenheit or thirty degrees Celsius) increase awakenings and reduce
slow-wave sleep. Some people are more sensitive to room temperature and other environmental conditions than others. If you find that
changes in room temperature interfere with your sleep, you should try
to maintain a constant temperature in your bedroom. Think of this as
another strategy for making your bedroom environment a cue for
sleeping. The precise temperature depends on you. Many people find
a cooler room more favorable for sleeping. If you can't afford an air
conditioner, try taking a hot shower before going to bed. After the
shower your body will cool and this will help you get to sleep faster.

Maintaining a low level of ambient noise is also important. If you happen to live in a noisy area, you should take steps to limit the amount of noise that reaches your bedroom (short of moving!). Keeping your windows closed can help. Having both blinds and drapes on your windows will filter out some of the noise (the heavy material of the drapes absorbs noises). You can also try to create a steady background noise ("white noise"), by using a fan or air conditioner to mask outside noises. On the other hand, the solution may be as simple as getting earplugs. If you use earplugs, however, make sure you can still hear your smoke or fire detector when wearing them.

Nearly everyone has a clock in his or her bedroom. That illuminated digital readout or the glowing hour and minute hands in the darkness can be a signal for anxiety in the typical insomniac. Many insomniacs will obsess over how much time has passed since they last looked at it. Persons with sleep problems frequently try to sleep on demand. You might go to bed at 11:00 and say to yourself, "Tonight I will fall asleep by 11:30 P.M., come hell or high water." Funny thing, however, the glances at the clock every ten minutes don't seem to help you fall asleep. You're now less sleepy than when you first got into bed.

You should try to make your bedroom a time-free zone. *Clock watching is one of the worst habits of the insomniac.* Once you see how much time has passed, it is hard to get it out of your head. Psychologist Daniel Wegner found that when people were given explicit instructions *not* to think of something (like a pink elephant for example), they found themselves doing the exact opposite. In fact, they found it difficult to get the image they were not supposed to think of out of their heads. A similar thing happens with clock-watching: once you check the clock a couple of times, it is difficult not to obsess about the sleep you are not getting. What's the solution? You still need an alarm clock to get you up at the same time every morning, but try setting the alarm and putting it under the bed or in the dresser drawer where it can still be reached when it goes off in the morning. This should prevent chronic, anxiety-inducing clock-watching.

Mattress quality is another important consideration in getting good sleep. Preference for mattress type and firmness differs from person to person. Among people with chronic back pain, however, there seems to be a consensus that *the firmer the better*. Waterbeds should generally be avoided. The size of the mattress can also affect your sleep quality, especially if you have a bed partner. When you sleep on a double (also called full-size) mattress with another person, you actually have less room than if you slept alone in a single or twin-size mattress. In fact, you each have about the same sleeping width as the average crib. Having extra room to move and shift positions without feeling as though you are disturbing your bed partner can be worth the expense of a larger mattress.

Best Sleeping Postures
Many people have asked about the best sleeping position to assume. If you have back pain, finding a comfortable position may be a challenge. The following are recommendations of physiotherapists.
• Lying on your side is preferable to lying on your stomach or back (especially if you have chronic back pain). Remember that you change positions when you sleep, so if you wake up on your stomach, then roll to your side or back.
• If you do sleep on your back, lie with your knees bent (put a pillow beneath them) to prevent stressing the back.
• Invest in a firm, high-quality pillow. Use only one pillow, tucked under your head and neck for support. Your pillow should be positioned so that it touches your shoulders. This is to prevent your head from being put into an unnatural position. Don't use two pillows! Your head and neck should be in an approximately straight line. Using two pillows raises your head above your shoulders and will create additional strain on your neck.
• Make effective and creative use of pillows to support other body parts (e.g. a pillow between legs when lying on the side takes strain off the back).
• Generally, mattresses that are neither too hard nor too soft are preferred by those with chronic pain. Newer design waterbeds (the waveless kind) provide more support than the older variety and are therefore better if you must have this type of bed. However, waterbeds can be difficult for some people to enter and exit.

- If you read in bed before sleep, use proper posture while sitting up in bed (i.e. don't read with your back flat and your head propped with pillows). It's actually best not to read in bed. Instead, read in a comfortable chair that provides neck and back support.
- Gentle stretching before bed is always a good practice.

Sleep Hygiene Recommendations

Product/ Practice	Effect on Sleep	Details	Recommendations
Caffeine	Negative	A central nervous system stimulant that enhances alertness.	Eliminate all caffeinated beverages after 6:00 P.M.
		More than two cups of coffee in the evening can increase time to fall asleep and cause more awakenings.	Heavy daytime consumers should cut down to less than four cups per day.
Nicotine	Negative	Another powerful stimulant.	Cut-down to less than one pack per day or quit altogether (professional assistance with smoking cessation is suggested).
		More than one pack per day increases time to fall asleep and causes awakenings.	
Alcohol	Negative	A central nervous system depressant that causes sleep fragmentation and early morning awakenings.	Avoid large amounts of alcohol, especially before bedtime.
Eating Habits	Negative	A large meal before sleep activates the digestive system and may cause awakenings.	Avoid large meals three to four hours before bed.
	Positive	As part of your presleep routine, a light snack before bedtime can promote sleep.	Have a small high carbohydrate snack (e.g., cheese and crackers) before bedtime.
Exercise	Positive	Increases slow-wave sleep, decreases time to fall asleep and reduces number of awakenings at night.	Do twenty to thirty minutes of mild to moderate exercise three three times per week (e.g., walking, cycling, swimming).
	Negative	Heavy exercise within two hours of bedtime stimulates your body and interferes with sleep.	Avoid any strenuous activities before bedtime.

chapter 15

WHERE DO I GO FROM HERE?: MAINTAINING TREATMENT GOALS

In this chapter you will:
- *Review your overall progress*
- *Learn how to cope with setbacks*

Be proud of yourself for getting this far. The program doesn't end here, however. This treatment is not like medication, which you take for a fixed period of time and then stop. You should continue with the skills you have learned in this program. It is important that you apply the skills and techniques on a continual basis to help you maintain a regular and satisfying sleep pattern. Think of it as an overall lifestyle change similar to maintaining a healthy diet. This book has shown you how to sleep the way most good sleepers do. It is up to you to maintain the progress you have made.

If, on the other hand, you did not achieve the goals you set out at the beginning of this book, retrace your steps and see which procedures you used and which you didn't. If you didn't use all the techniques, especially the good sleep habits guidelines in chapter 7, then you should go back and try others. Remember that not everyone responds to the techniques at the same rate, so give it time.

If you avoid or skip regular practice of these strategies and your sleep quality is still unsatisfactory, ask yourself why you chose not to do the work. Make sure you give yourself a good reason, because ultimately you are in charge of your own self-management program. A

common reason people give themselves for not using or learning a
new skill is that it is too hard for them to change old habits or they are
too busy with other activities to put the skill into practice. If this is
your reason, then ask yourself:

How important is quality sleep to me?
How much longer can I endure my poor quality sleep?
Are these other activities more important than my sleep quality?

If you answered yes to the last question, then you have made
the decision to sacrifice your efforts at achieving good sleep to other
needs and interests. Is this wise?

If you answered no, then ask yourself: Why are these other
activities taking priority? What needs are served by devoting my energy
to these activities instead of working to improve my sleep quality?

Ultimately, you are responsible for your continued success.
You now have the knowledge and skills to make your sleep better, so
you should not feel like the passive victim of your sleep problem.

Motivating Yourself to Continue
Achieving better sleep will probably be the best motivation you can
find for continuing to practice your :60 Second sleep-ease skills.

In addition, it may help to self-monitor your sleep periodically
to remind yourself of how well you are sleeping. For example, every
six months you could fill out the sleep log for a two to three week
period and then chart your progress. Use this as an opportunity to
identify areas of drift in your sleep pattern that may have occurred
since finishing the program. For example, are you still maintaining a
regular rising time? Do you restrict your time in bed to no more than
one hour greater than the total time you are sleeping? Remember that
it is normal to have the occasional night of bad sleep. It is important
to look at your overall sleep pattern using two to three weeks of self-
monitoring as your source of information.

Coping with Setbacks
It is important to be able to recognize when you are having a setback
or "relapse" back to bad sleep. Remember that one or two nights of

poor sleep is not a relapse since most people have occasional nights of troubled sleep. Of course, you are the best judge as to whether you are falling into a pattern of chronic insomnia again. If your previous poor sleep pattern emerges again for at least two weeks, then you should take some steps to correct it.

Make sure that any setback in your sleep pattern is not related to a new stressor in your life or change in your health status. Some questions to ask yourself are:

- Is there a new personal or financial stressor in my life now (for example, change in income, marriage/divorce/separation, loss of a loved one, moving or change in living arrangements)?
- Have I been feeling more depressed or anxious than usual? Can I identify the reason why?
- Am I taking any new medications?
- Have I started drinking more than usual?
- Am I smoking too much or drinking too much coffee or caffeinated beverages?

Disturbed sleep can be a symptom of any of these reasons, so rule them out as possible causal factors before proceeding with a relapse plan. To be on the safe side, report any sudden and dramatic change in your sleep to your physician. If it is related to a change in your health, you can still use your relapse plan to make your sleep better; just ensure that the primary problem is also being treated.

The first thing to remember about a relapse is not to panic. Relapses are normal and expected. Don't let yourself become overwhelmed with negative self-defeating thoughts. On the other hand, you shouldn't ignore a relapse and hope that it goes away on its own. If anything, a relapse is just a reminder that your condition requires ongoing management. A relapse should be a learning opportunity, not a personal failure.

One of the best ways to cope with a relapse is to have a plan prepared beforehand. The plan will be personal and depend on your preferences for sleep improving techniques and coping strategies. You can make your work easier by knowing ahead of time what your strengths and weaknesses are. If your relapse is related to one of these weaknesses, then the first step may be to go back and read the relevant chapter. You don't have to read the whole book again, just the chapters relevant to your relapse.

Make a new list that will be your relapse plan. You can include any skill or set of skills from the manual. Put them in order of priority and expected effectiveness. An example of a plan for coping with a relapse is provided below. As a suggestion, the first three in this list should also be in your relapse plan, preferably at the top as well.

1. Follow *all* the stimulus control guidelines to the letter, not just the ones that worked for you. (chapter 7)
2. Make sure your time in bed never exceeds your total time sleeping by more than one hour. Use the sleep restriction method to improve this. (chapter 6)
3. Read chapter 10 to remind yourself of the dangers of negative self-talk about sleep.
4. Don't cut back on any daytime activities, especially pleasurable ones just because of poor sleep.
5. Avoid napping during the day; try to keep busy with mentally challenging tasks; avoid boring or mentally passive activities such as watching television.
6. Be more physically active during the day to increase deep sleep at night.
7. Use positive reaffirming self-talk:
    "Insomnia will go away."
    'I coped with it before, I can cope with it again."
    "I have the skills now to help me get through this."
8. Tell your spouse/friends about your condition to elicit their support and understanding.

On the next page is a blank relapse prevention plan with a few reminders for good sleeping habits.

Good luck and good night!

What I Should Do if My Sleep Becomes Unsatisfactory Again: A Relapse Prevention Plan

Strategy to use	Chapter to read
1._____	
Example: Get out of bed when unable to sleep	7
2._____	
Example: Don't spend excess time in bed	6
3._____	
Example: Cut out caffeine and alcohol in the evening	14
4._____	
5._____	
6._____	
7._____	
8._____	

ENDNOTES

CHAPTER 2

1. S. Ancoli-Israel & T. Roth, (1999). "Characteristics of Insomnia in the United States: Results of the 1991 National Sleep Foundation Survey," *Sleep* 22, Suppl. 2 (1999): 347-353.
2. L. Dotto, *Losing Sleep* (New York: William Morrow and Company, 1990).
3. Ibid.
4. G.K. Zammit, et al., "Quality of Life in People with Insomnia." *Sleep* 22, Suppl. 2 (1999): 379-385.
5. J.K. Walsh & C.L. Engelhardt, "The Direct Economic Costs of Insomnia in the United States for 1995," *Sleep* 22, Suppl. 2 (1999): 386-393.

CHAPTER 3

1. H. Tait, "Sleep Problems: Whom Do They Affect?" *Statistics Canada: Canadian Social Trends* (Winter 1992): 8-10.
2. S.R. Currie, et al., "Cognitive-behavioral Treatment of Insomnia Secondary to Chronic Pain," *Journal of Consulting and Clinical Psychology* 68 (2000).
3. T. Roehrs, et al., "Ethanol as a hypnotic in insomniacs: Self-administration and effects on sleep and mood," *Neuropsychopharmacology* 20 (1999): 279-286.
4. D.L. Bliwise, "Normal Aging" in M.H. Kryger, et al., *Principles and Practice of Sleep Medicine* (Philadelphia: Saunders, 2000): 26-42.
5. C.M. Morin, et al., "Behavioral and Pharmacological Therapies for Late-life Insomnia: a Randomized Controlled Trial," *Journal of the American Medical Association* 281 (1998): 991-999.

CHAPTER 12
1. J.L.F. Shaver & S.N. Zenk, "Sleep disturbance in menopause," *Journal of Women's Health & Gender-based Medicine* 9 (2000): 109-118.
2. R. Manber & R. Armitage, "Sex steroids and sleep: A review," *Sleep* 22 (1999): 540-555.
3. M.T. Anarte, J.L. Cuadros & J. Herrera, "Hormonal and psychological treatments: therapeutic alternative for menopausal women," *Maturitas* 29 (1998): 203-208.
4. Shaver, "Sleep Disturbance in Menopause," 109-118.

CHAPTER 13
1. J.A. Mindell, "Sleep Disorders in Children." *Health Psychology* 12 (1993): 151-162.
2. A. Eisenberg, H.E. Murkoff & S.E. Hathaway, *What to Expect the First Year,* (New York: Workman Publishing, 1996).
3. G. Stores, "Practitioner review: Assessment and Treatment of Sleep Disorders in Children and Adolescents," *Journal of Child Psychology and Psychiatry* 37 (1996): 907-925.
4. K.L. Maelstrom & C.M. Freeman, "School Start Time Study: Report Summary," University of Minnesota: The Center for Applied Research and Educational Improvement, College of Education and Human Development (1997).
5. National Sleep Foundation Sleep and Teens Task Force, *Adolescent Sleep Needs and Patterns: Research Report and Resource guide,* Washington: National Sleep Foundation (2000).
6. A.I. Pack, et al., "Characteristics of Crashes Attributed to the Driver Having Fallen Asleep," *Accident Analysis & Prevention* 27 (1995): 769-775.

CHAPTER 14
1. P. Tiffin, et al., "Pharmacokinetic and Pharamacodynamic Responses to Caffeine in Poor and Normal Sleepers," *Psychopharamacology* 121 (1995): 494-502.
2. F. Lexcen & R. Hick, "Does Cigarette Smoking Increase Sleep Problems?" *Perceptual & Motor Skills* 77 (1994): 16-18.
3. A. Fugh-Berman & J.M. Cott, "Dietary Supplements and Natural Products as Psychotherapeutic Agents," *Psychosomatic Medicine* 61 (1999): 712-728.

RESOURCES ON SLEEP AND HEALTH

Information on Sleep Disorders

American Sleep Apnea Association
1424 K Street NW, Suite 302
Washington, DC 20005
(202) 293-3650 • fax: (202) 29303656
Web site: http://www.sleepapnea.org • E-mail: asaa@sleepapnea.org
A non-profit organization that promotes awareness of sleep apnea.

National Sleep Foundation
1522 K Street NW, Suite 500
Washington, DC 20005
(202) 347-3471 • fax: (202) 347-3472
Web site: http://www.sleepfoundation.org • E-mail: NSF@sleepfoundation.org
A national non-profit organization dedicated to improving the lives of
millions of Americans who suffer from sleep disorders.

Restless Legs Syndrome Foundation, Inc.
P.O. Box 7050 or 819 Second Street, SW
Rochester, MN 55902
Web site: http://www.rls.org • E-mail: RLSFoundation@rls.org
Dedicated to increasing awareness, developing effective treatments and
finding a cure for Restless Legs Syndrome.

SleepNet
Web site: http://www.sleepnet.com.
An interactive web site with current information on a variety of sleep
topics including sleep disorders.

Books on Chronic Pain
:60 Second Chronic Pain Relief by Peter G. Lehndorff, M.D., with Brian Tarcy, (Far Hills, NJ: New Horizon Press, 1997).
Managing Pain Before it Manages You by Margaret Caudill (Toronto: Guilford Press, 1996).
Managing Back Pain: Self-Help Manual by Michael S. Melnick, et al. (Chaska, Minnesota: The Saunders Group, 1989).

Self-Help Books
:60 Second Stress Management by Dr. Andrew Goliszek (Far Hills, NJ: New Horizon Press, 1992).
The Relaxation & Stress Reduction Workbook, Fourth Edition by Martha Davis (Oakland, CA: New Harbinger Publications, 1995).
The Feeling Good Handbook by David Burns (Toronto: Penguin Books, 1989).
:60 Second Menopause Management by Carol Schultz and Mary Jenkins, MD, (Far Hills, NJ: New Horizon Press, 1996).
:60 Second Mind/Body Rejuvenation by Curtis Turchin, D.C., M.A. (Far Hills, NJ: New Horizon Press, 2000).

Alcohol and Drug Resources

Alcoholics Anonymous – World Services
Grand Central Station
P.O. Box 459
New York, NY 10163
Web site: http://www.aa.org

Narcotics Anonymous – World Services
P.O. Box 9999
Van Nuys, California 91409
(818) 773-9999 • fax (818) 700-0700
Web site: http://www.na.org

Quitting Smoking Web Sites:
http://quitnet.org
http://www.lungusa.org
http://www.drkoop.com/wellness/tobacco

KNOWLEDGE QUIZ

Each of the questions has one answer that is better than all of the others. Please circle the letter beside the answer that you think is best. Try to answer all the questions even if you have to guess. An answer key with explanations follows the quiz.

1. Insomnia is most often caused by _____.
   (a) pain
   (b) a chemical imbalance
   (c) performance anxiety
   (d) growing old

2. Why is slow-wave (deep) sleep important?
   (a) It is the stage of sleep where dreaming takes place.
   (b) It is the most restful stage of sleep for the body and mind.
   (c) It helps to regulate temperature.
   (d) It helps the immune system fight illness.

3. You can possibly increase the amount of deep sleep you have at night by _____.
   (a) making sure not to nap during the daytime
   (b) taking vitamins
   (c) avoiding physical activity after 5:00 p.m.
   (d) going to bed early

178 :60 Second Sleep-Ease

4. Which of the following is not an effective way of coping with chronic sleep problems?
   (a) avoiding daytime napping
   (b) getting up at the same time every morning
   (c) going to bed only when you are tired
   (d) staying in bed until sleep finally comes

5. The best thing to do when you have a poor night's sleep is to
   (a) take a nap during the day to recover the lost sleep
   (b) go to bed earlier the following night
   (c) reduce your activities for the day
   (d) go to bed at the same time you normally would

6. Wanting to sleep as well as you did when you were eighteen is an example of _____.
   (a) an unrealistic expectation
   (b) the power of positive thinking
   (c) low self-esteem
   (d) a self-fulfilling prophesy

7. Which of the following is the most important condition for falling asleep?
   (a) putting your body in a state of relaxation
   (b) a cool room temperature
   (c) putting your mind in a relaxed state
   (d) a firm, comfortable mattress

8. One good thing to do when you can't get to sleep is to _____.
   (a) get out of bed and read a boring book
   (b) do some exercise to feel tired
   (c) drink some hot chocolate
   (d) take some medication

9. To avoid interference with your sleep, you should not drink any caffeinated beverages _____.
   (a) one hour before bedtime
   (b) two hours before bedtime
   (c) three to four hours before bedtime
   (d) more than four hours before bedtime

10. Clock-watching when trying to fall asleep is bad because _____.
    (a) the time seems to go by so slowly
    (b) you often misread the time on a digital clock when very tired
    (c) it increases your focus on the fact that you are not sleeping
    (d) it can be a strain on your neck

11. Which of the following is not a good pre-bedtime activity?
    (a) taking a hot bath
    (b) having a glass of warm milk
    (c) doing the household finances
    (d) imagery relaxation

12. Most sleeping pills help you sleep by giving you more _____.
    (a) dreams
    (b) light sleep
    (c) deep sleep
    (d) a and b

13. If you have to nap, the best time to do it is in the _____.
    (a) late afternoon
    (b) morning
    (c) early evening
    (d) mid-afternoon

14. Believing that you need eight hours of sleep each and every night is an example of _____.
    (a) emotional reasoning
    (b) catastrophizing
    (c) goal-setting
    (d) all-or-nothing thinking

15. Which of the following is not a good way to reduce stressful thoughts before bedtime?
    (a) imagining a pleasant scene in your mind
    (b) telling yourself not to worry
    (c) writing down your problems on paper
    (d) thinking about the worst that could happen and then developing a coping plan

16. Sleep efficiency is _____.
    (a) a measure of how fast you can fall asleep
    (b) the ratio of your good nights of sleep to bad nights in a typical
         week
    (c) the ratio of your hours spent sleeping to hours spent in bed
    (d) a measure of how deep your sleep is

17. In general, the time you spend in bed should not exceed the time you
    spend sleeping by more than _____.
    (a) three hours
    (b) two hours
    (c) one hour
    (d) twenty minutes

18. Which of the following is the best way to exercise if you want to sleep
    better?
    (a) a brisk walk every day at the same time
    (b) twenty minutes of intense aerobic exercise once or twice per week
    (c) change the exercise depending on the season (e.g., skating in the
         winter, swimming in the summer)
    (d) choose individual over group or paired sports

19. Lying in bed at night thinking about your problems or sleep loss can
    lead to _____.
    (a) an association forming between your bed and anxiety
    (b) a solution to some of your problems if you lie there long enough
    (c) an increase in the use of sleeping medications
    (d) a headache

20. The best way to avoid napping during the daytime is to _____.
    (a) find an activity to do outside your home
    (b) drink coffee to stay awake
    (c) read a book or watch television
    (d) take a cold shower

Answer Key:

1. c. Pain and getting old can contribute to insomnia, however, performance anxiety is the most common cause of sleep problems in chronic insomniacs.
2. b.
3. a. Napping can rob you of your nighttime deep sleep.
4. d. Trying to force yourself to sleep contributes to performance anxiety.
5. d. The other choices will only reinforce your belief that a single bad night is catastrophic.
6. a. Sleep needs very depending on age; it is unrealistic to expect that you will sleep as well as when you were younger.
7. c. The other choices certainly contiribute to better sleep but without having your mind in a relaxed state, none of them will make much of a difference.
8. a. You should choose activities that are not physically or mentally stimulating when you are trying to fall asleep.
9. d. Caffeine takes a long time (up to seven hours) to clear your body.
10. c. If you find yourself clock-watching, move the alarm clock to a location within reach but hidden out of sight (e.g. drawer of a bedside table).
11. c. Doing any activity before bedtime that increases stress or anxiety can disturb your sleep.
12. b. Most benzodiazepine medications increase total sleep time at the expense of time spent in deep sleep.
13. b. Napping in the afternoons or later is equivalent to starting your nighttime deep sleep before even going to bed.
14. d. Not everyone needs eight hours of sleep every night. The average needed for adults is between four and ten hours. Quality sleep is better than quantity.
15. b. Telling yourself not to worry and doing nothing else can increase your anxiety.
16. c. See page 43 for a definition of and more information on sleep efficiency.
17. c.
18. a. Regular daily exercise is better than bursts of intense exercise.
19. a.
20. a.

Name: _____

SLEEP LOG for the week of _____ to _____

	SUN.	MON.	TUES.	WED.	THURS.	FRI.	S_
To be completed in the evening							
1. Did you take any naps today? (Y = Yes, N = No) If yes, give total length in minutes.							
2. How many cups of caffeinated coffee did you drink today?							
3. How many cups of caffeinated tea (i.e. not herbal) did you drink today?							
4. How many cigarettes did you smoke today?							
To be completed in the morning							
1. What time did you go to bed? (A.M./P.M.?)							
2. What time did you get out of bed? (A.M./P.M.?)							
3. Approximately how many hours of sleep did you get last night (to the nearest half hour)?							
4. How long did it take you to fall asleep?							
5. How many times did you wake up during the night?							
6. In the morning did you awaken at the time you wanted to? (E = Earlier, O = On time, L = Later)							
7. Rate the overall quality of your sleep (0 = Extremely Poor to 5 = Extremely Good)							
8. Rate how rested you felt this morning upon awakening (0 = Not at all Rested to 5 = Well Rested)							

$$\text{Sleep Efficiency} = \frac{\text{Total Sleep Time [\#3]}}{\text{Time Spent in Bed}} \times 100$$

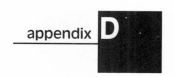

SELF-MANAGEMENT VERSUS SLEEPING PILLS

Self-management	Sleeping Pills
Take control of own sleeping behavior (**ACTIVE** treatment)	No control; you are dependent on the pills to do all the work (**PASSIVE** treatment)
More effective in long-term control of sleep disturbances (research to back this up)	Pills lose their effectiveness after two to three weeks of use at constant dosage
Doesn't lead to addiction	Can become addicted (physically dependent on the drug so that your body constantly needs the drug)
No side-effects	Side-effects: daytime drowsiness, alertness and performance at psychomotor tasks (e.g., driving) impaired, memory difficulties, "hangover" feeling
No health dangers involved	Health dangers: risk to fetus if taken during pregnancy; risk of overdose if combined with alcohol or other drugs
Under right circumstances, will increase valuable slow-wave and REM sleep	Most sleeping pills reduce slow-wave and REM sleep
No risk of tolerance; actually, opposite generally occurs: your sleep gets better with continued application	Tolerance builds with prolonged use
Low risk of rebound insomnia effects	Rebound insomnia can occur with sudden discontinuation of pills
Free	Expensive ($$)

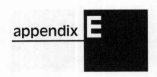

MY PROGRESS CHARTS

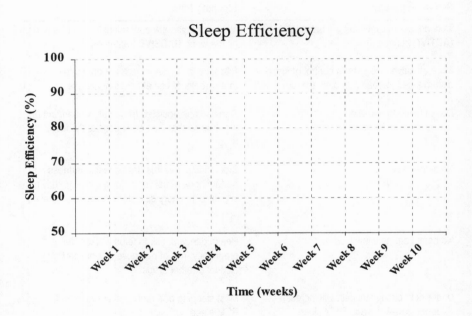

Sleep Efficiency

Sleep Quality

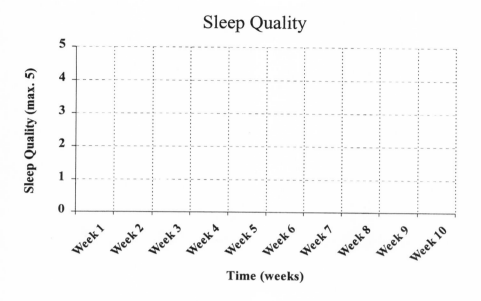

Time to Fall Asleep

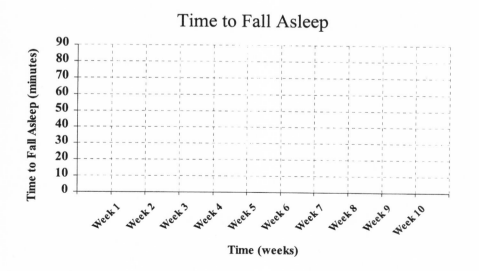

Number of Awakenings

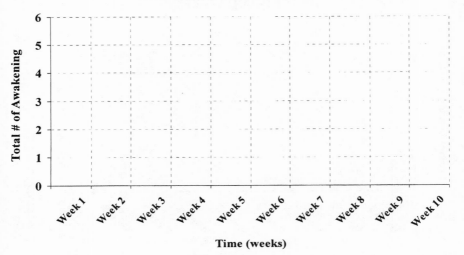

Time (weeks)

Other Titles in the :60 Second Series